You, Me & PSP

By Steve Dagnell

Printed and bound in England by www.printondemand-worldwide.com

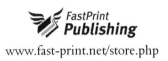

www.fast-print.net/store.php

You, Me & PSP
Copyright © Steve Dagnell 2016

A catalogue record for this book is available from the British Library

ISBN 978-178456-396-7

First published 2016 by
FASTPRINT PUBLISHING
Peterborough, England.

Foreword

By
Field Marshal the Lord Guthrie of Craigiebank
GCB, LVO, OBE, DL
President of the PSP Association

Cilla Dagnell had a passion for life and love. An energetic and flamboyant character, she filled her days with adventure and laughter, fun and friendship.

Sadly, her life was to be cruelly cut short following a diagnosis of progressive supranuclear palsy (PSP), a devastating and incurable neurological condition.

PSP would slowly and brutally rob Cilla of the ability to walk, talk, see and swallow. But it would not take away her sharpness of mind or strength of spirit.

'You, Me & PSP' is an honest, open and often humorous account of Cilla's fascinating and colourful world, both before and while living with PSP.

We first get to know the young Cilla, a busy, energetic and fun-loving child who loved animals and rubbed shoulders with stars of music, stage and screen.

As an adult, flirtatious Cilla was the life and soul of the party, much loved for her spontaneity, charm, wit and infectious laughter.

But sadly her life was to change dramatically. A period of unexplained illnesses finally 'made sense' when she was eventually diagnosed with PSP. It was shattering news for Cilla and her husband Steve.

Page by page, Cilla and Steve selflessly take us through the physical symptoms and emotional impact of PSP, so that we may learn from their experiences.

Despite new daily challenges, numerous medical appointments and an increasing reliance on others, Cilla never made a fuss. Her cherished friendships remained firm to the end as is fondly recounted in touching tales of her raucous laughter and storytelling with 'the girls'.

'Never in a million years could I ever imagined myself in the role of carer...' Steve shares his innermost feelings as he strives to balance his unfolding role of carer, with that of husband. He ensured that his wife's most personal and medical needs were fully met, and her nails and hair were always maintained to her usual high standard!

Thanks to the devoted couple's openness throughout the book, many families affected by PSP will no doubt find comfort in their reflections, alongside practical information on issues such as communication, feeding and planning for the future.

'You, Me & PSP' does not shy away from difficult topics: Cilla was adamant they should be included. Neither does it attempt to give advice. Instead it shares hints, tips and information drawn from personal experience.

Cilla was a prolific diarist and blogger and many of the words in this book are her own. 'You, Me & PSP' was mostly written during Cilla's lifetime and, when no longer able to speak, she gave Steve's words her approval with a 'thumbs up'.

Generous to the end, Cilla wanted others affected by PSP to benefit from this book. Proceeds are being donated to the PSP Association (PSPA), the only national charity in the UK that provides information and support for those affected by PSP while funding research into the condition.

Sadly, Cilla passed away in 2015. But she will not be forgotten. You, Me & PSP is a touching and fitting legacy through which her memory lives on.

SUPPORTED BY

Mr & Mrs Mark Roberts, Ann Weakley

Mr Thomas Vail, and the combined Vail and Eastwood Families in memory of Mr John Vail who sadly passed away from complications due to PSP in March 2013

~

Jonathan Terry, Independent Funeral Directors

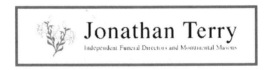

Alyson Roach
Alyson@bnihampshire.com

Executive Director
+44 (0)7989 320893

To maximise funding from the proceeds of this book, it was felt that self-publishing was the way forward since this method eliminated certain third parties and their associated fees. Based on that logic, every last penny from sales of this book through the PSP Association and other outlets is going directly into their coffers in the name of Cilla Dagnell.

It shows true worth to support an author... but it shows exceptional worth to financially support an author who has written so passionately about a little known illness such as PSP and the human element behind it.

In this instance, the author – and all of those connected through the all-embracing network involved with PSP – would like to express their absolute gratitude to all of the aforementioned for their unprecedented financial support in making this eventuality possible.

Together, we have worked tirelessly to produce a book full of love, fervour, empathy, positivity, human endurance and, unfortunately, sadness. Combine this and you get an individual perspective of what it is like to live with an unrelenting disease such as PSP.

As a reader, you too have chosen to support the PSP Association, since *ALL* proceeds from the sales of this book are being donated for the next twenty-five years.

Ultimately, with your help and that of our main sponsors, we aim to challenge PSP head-on and find a method of treating the illness or even eliminating it for good!

In Memory of
John Williams
02.01.1950 – 28.02.2015
&
Thomas Bengtsson
06.09.1954 – 14.02.2016

~

In loving memory of Peter Andow
who sadly passed 03.06.16

~

To all our loved ones present and passed
It won't be long, so hold on fast
Free from pain and free from strife
You left behind a broken life

Yet you have proven that we must go
Leaving behind a trail of woe
But if truth be told, and we all agree
It's not that bad to be this free

Memories now we hold so dear
And with you waiting we hold no fear
So we'll be along at our own pace
To look upon your smiling face

So, please save me a seat by your side
But before you do, be my guide
And help me through these last dark days
By leading me through the eternal rays

Steve Dagnell

Our time on Earth is but a blink
Sometimes not enough to think
And through those left upon their wake
Memories of their lives we make
So think often of those gone by
And never let their memories die!

Steve Dagnell

With Thanks to the Following for Their Invaluable Services to Cilla Over the Years

<u>Carers (In Alphabetical order)</u>
<u>2013-2015</u>

Abby Waterhouse, Alex Wilkinson, Anita Baker, Arlene Moody, Beverly Slight, Bid Norris, Bobbie Ribeiro, Chrissy Calder, Clare Freemantle, Dale-Anne Bevan, Dawn Stansbridge, Donna Coe, Edit Halaszne Ronai, Ellie Lee, Emma Agboola, Georgie Huskins, Hannah Foster, Hannah Ramsey, Heidi Lloyd, Helen Craddock, Jenna Bright, Karen Dancey, Karen Orchard, Kate Haines, Katie Green, Katie McLaren, Kay Monckton, Kelly Webb, Kerrie Potter, Kerry Pullinger, Kim Green, Kirsty Darcy, Kirsty Howes, Laura Wilson, Lisa Beever, Liz Saunders, Lou Simmons, Lucy Downes, Mandy Cull, Maria Pop, Naomi Gibbs, Pauline Barnett, Rachael Crosby, Rose Jones, Sarah Sleeman, Shannon Darcy, Stacey Humphrey, Theresa Porter, Zoë Millington

<u>Carers – Special Mention</u>

Bobbie Ribeiro, Naomi Gibbs
Rose Jones,
Stacey Humphrey

<u>Carers – Beyond the Call of Duty</u>

Georgie Huskins, Hannah Foster,
Kerrie Potter

Special Mention

Kerry Brady (Mayflower Theatre Southampton)

-

Dave & Paulene Landsey

-

Special Contribution

Niki Browes & Family

Daily Mail OnLine

http://www.dailymail.co.uk/home/index.html

Medical Professionals

Dr Olivia Rodrigues MBBS, MRCGP
(*West End Surgery Southampton*)
Dr Ashwin Pinto MA BM BCh FRCP DPhil
(*Consultant Neurologist Winchester*)
Dr Alice Manson MBBS, MRCP
(*Consultant Neurologist Winchester*)
Dr Boyd Ghosh MA, MBBS, PhD Clinical
Neuroscience, MRCP
Dr Andrew Jenks MBBS, MRCP, MSc
(*Countess Mountbatten Hospice*)
Dr Anna Hume MBBS, MSc
(*Countess Mountbatten Hospice*)
Anna Mills (*McDonald*) Speech & Therapy OT
(*Adult Mental Health, Hamble*)
District Nurses
(*Integrated Community Care Team, Eastleigh*)
Dr Emily Heiden & Team
(*Ward D5, Southampton General Hospital*)

Social Service & Advisors

Marion Wells (Adult Social Services H C C)
Samantha Griffiths (Adult Social Services H C C)
Wendy Symons (Adult Social Services H C C)
Jenny Kilroy (Adult Social Services H C C)
Jenny Webb OT (Eastleigh Borough Council)
Hampshire C C Equipment & Delivery Service
Red Cross/Solent Healthcare NHS
Wessex Housing Association

PSP Association

http://www.pspassociation.org.uk/

Louisa Roberts-West (Hampshire Local PSPA Group)
Fergus Logan (Chief Executive PSPA)
Paula McGrath (Director of Communications PSPA)
Cameron Wood (Director of Development PSPA)
Peter Daniels (Director of Information and Support PSPA)
Kathy Weston (Specialist Care Advisor PSPA)
Jane Stein (Specialist Care Advisor PSPA)

Contributions (In Alphabetical Order)

Adrian Dagnell, Amy Brand
Andy Tierney, Ann Raynor
Dr Suzy Shuttleworth MBBS
Georgie Huskins, Hannah Foster
Jez Hadlow, Joan Roberts
Muna Roberts-Bond, Joe Upson
Mary Lawrence, Nigel Pope
Paul & Jill Upson, Peter Dagnell
Robin & Liz Alsford

<u>Useful Addresses & Internet Links</u>

For Both PSP & CBD
PSP Association
PSP House
167 Watling Street West
Towcester, Northamptonshire, NN12 6BX
Tel: UK +44 (0)1327 322410
Email: psp@pspassociation.org.uk/

-

Helpline advisers provide a confidential telephone and email service offering information, practical and emotional support to people living with PSP and http://klo.io/1JE7Wwh helpline@pspassociation.org.uk or phone, Monday to Friday, between 9am-5pm and 7-9pm.
http://bit.ly/1nQJ0c6

-

Facebook:
https://www.facebook.com/PSPAssociation

-

General PSP Questions Answered
http://www.psp.org/education/faq.html

-

Queen Square Brain Bank for Neurological Disorders
University College London
Gower Street
London WC1E 6BT
Tel: UK +44 (0)20 7679 2000
http://www.ucl.ac.uk/contact-list/

-

Parkinson's UK
http://www.parkinsons.org.uk/
Helpline: 0808 800 0303

-

Care Quality Commission
http://www.cqc.org.uk/
Tel: 03000 616161

Steve Dagnell

With Heartfelt Thanks

A s an author, I hold three things very dear. Firstly, the developing story; secondly, my readers and their needs; but above all and finally, my editor.

The sequence above is not an accident, since without the story I would not have the readers; but no matter how good the story is, it would not please the eye if it were peppered with errors - grammatical or otherwise.

Therefore, I am delighted to have had the professional services of Kimberley L Humphries, who has, in this instance, given her time and expertise at no expense in the cause to raise the awareness of PSP.

For me to fully get my message across I needed complete trust in both the proofing and editing. Certainly, with Kimberley's selfless assistance in this matter, I feel the end product is a polished and candid insight into this complex illness.

I honestly cannot think of a better tribute to Cilla than what you are about to read.

Kimberley, I thank you from the bottom of my heart.

Kimberley L Humphries

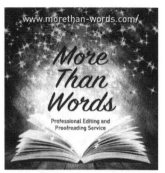

more than words
professional editing and proofreading service

UK landline: 01788 824577
UK mobile: 07754 778910
www.morethan-words.com/
www.linkedin.com/profile/

'To my friend and fellow author, Steve,

Thank you for the privilege and honour of editing 'You, Me & PSP'. What a beautiful and fabulous woman Cilla was, adored by you and by all who met her. Her magic shines in your words, her spirit dances.

In penning this incredible story of indomitable human spirit and love, you have fulfilled a promise to Cilla, and the world will thank you for your determination, and Cilla's, to reach out to all those encountering PSP.

Kimberley'

With Heartfelt Thanks

W hen I first became an author I was made aware, by others, that the publishing business was cut throat and for me to be prepared for some nasty surprises. Cautiously, and with naïve trepidation I forged ahead. After all, I was inspired and prompted by Cilla to write... and this is now her legacy.

After publishing my first two novels, I awaited the inevitable downfall and the associated un-pleasantries... but they never came. Whether I chose my associates well, or the initial information I was first given was false, I have been blessed with nothing but help and kindness.

As you already know, there are those who have helped beyond expectations and as I delved into the unknown world of ebooks I found another.

Colin Timms founder and creator of The Electronic Book Company, produced my third novel, 'One for Rose Cottage' in ebook form for me. Not only did he do this but he advised me all the way. Indeed, the book in both forms is a success thanks partly to his input. So, it would not surprise you to know that I once more approached him to produce the ebook version of *You, Me & PSP*. It was a surprise to me though, that Colin had anticipated my call, and before I could talk to him about the project, he said, *"I know about Cilla and I am sorry to hear of your loss. I understand that you would like to produce an e version of her life story. Not a problem since it is for charity, I shall make no charge and do what I can."*

I was dumbfounded and stunned by his gracious offer of help, which I gratefully accepted.

It is with utmost respect that I offer this small offering as a thank you Colin for your kindness and help in my time of reflection. Colin Timms, you are a true gentleman.

Ann & Rod Raynor

A dear friend named Ann Raynor sadly lost her husband Rod to PSP and was, due to her association with the illness, offered the opportunity to read a final draft of 'You, Me & PSP'. She was then given a chance to express her full and honest opinion, which, with her permission, reads as follows:

'I have just finished reading yours and Cilla's story.

At the moment I am lost for words and feeling very emotional - It is a beautiful story.

I would love to have met Cilla a woman with a zest for life, she knew what she wanted from life and what Cilla wanted Cilla got.

It was good to get know Cilla before she was cruelly struck with PSP... and you my friend well what can I say, the way you cared for her, loved her, reminds me of the wonderful love Rod and I shared together.

Your story is going help a lot of people . . . you have gone into great detail as regarding to PSP, it is quite emotional to read.

Everyone will enjoy getting to know Cilla at the beginning of the book.

'You, Me & PSP' is going to be a great success and I know Cilla will be smiling down on you and feeling so proud of you.'

In loving memory of Rod Raynor – From his beloved Wife Ann

You, Me & PSP

Steve Dagnell

Introduction

As an author, Steve Dagnell – aka Shelby Locke – has specific aims. Under normal circumstances he wants to get his work out there and into the public domain as quickly as possible. With research done, the story written, layouts and editing are constants until finally – to the publishing house before reaching bookshelves, e-books and other sales outlets.

In Shelby Locke's words: *'It is all about the story!'*

This story is, however, significantly different from anything he has previously written. Why? Because it is a story he did not want to finish. And by finishing this story, he is in essence, telling you that the person he is writing about, loved and cared for over many years – his dear wife Cilla – has died.

Due to the multiplicity of the subject, this book is in several sections and has no chapters, just headings. The story dictates absolute dedication to the human element, which is so important to everyone concerned in Cilla's life. After all, the book could just as well be referring to anybody suffering from this illness, or any other illness that remotely resembles its symptoms.

It was also felt by the author that by reading this that you, the reader, would understand the full and final impact of the story and continue to ponder on its content well beyond the closing words...

Sadly, as of the early hours of Wednesday 16th of December 2015, and through grief-stricken eyes, the story thus started.

You, Me & PSP

So why the title, I hear you ask? The answer is quite simple really: it evolved!

You... This is specifically designed for you: the reader, relative, carer, sufferer, newly diagnosed sufferer, or just an interested party committed to learn about this unusual illness. It is also intended to help you understand PSP from a long-term sufferer's point of view.

The term **Me...** relates to Cilla, a sixty-six-year-old wife, mother, grandmother and PSP sufferer. And, of course, there is the human side of everything to do with her life before and leading up to the hereafter. Logically, once you understand PSP, then you will realise that there is no way on earth that Cilla could have written this book, since PSP has precluded her from that ability. Therefore, it has been, with her selfless help, left for me to write on her behalf.

& PSP... the illness that has so mercilessly taken her life and the cruel, interminable way it finally took it.

It was thought at first that the story could be told whilst Cilla was still alive. However, due to the diversity and speed of the illness, especially in the latter stages of her life with PSP, it was thought best by all concerned to wait until the very end; this reflection included Cilla's own feelings.

What you are about to read is a true account of Cilla's life up until now – today. Or, because of the illnesses complexities – today's yesterdays.

This book will also offer a small amount of practical guidance to all carers involved in the illness, mainly through experience, but also through the eyes of the sufferer.

Since Cilla's brain remained intact throughout the whole term – despite being locked inside her body – and whilst she had full understanding, she was continually consulted throughout this labour of love. Her approval was frequently sought, and thumbs-up were quite literally given as a sign to proceed.

Equally, Cilla believed that this book should only financially benefit those with PSP and therefore felt that all proceeds should be donated to the PSP Association; her wish, along with many other wishes associated with her illness, have unequivocally been granted.

You

PSP might not even be applicable to you. Indeed, it might not even be on your radar. But there is one thing we share for certain: finality!

It is how you deal with this finality that makes what I have to say so pertinent to you.

You. Yes, you – the reader.

I want you to completely appreciate that the person involved in this book is real. The facts speak for themselves and, more importantly, are as accurate as I can possibly relate them. To fully understand this point then please read on.

By the end of the book, I want you to be able to close your eyes and visualise Cilla as a young girl, through her teens, and beyond. To understand the zest for life from within, and to enjoy her sense of humour, as well as her ability to make others happy.

I also want you to understand this: Cilla was once a much-loved daughter, a little girl, a sister, a friend, a girlfriend, a wife and a grandmother; so many roles to play in life's daily merry-go-round, yet all encompassed in one person. I point this out because when we see someone of her age group dying, we tend to forget this fact. We, as humans, seem to overlook the fact that we all once had a childhood filled with vigour, expectations and a fearless approach to the future. Son or daughter, *YOU* are no different to Cilla, and the process of life affects us all.

So from now on, I need you to open your minds and absorb what I... no, correction... *we* as a couple, have to tell you.

Overview

Incidentally, when I said earlier 'locked inside her body' I mean just that. And when I say 'dead'... well, there is no easy way of saying it other than what it is, since there is currently no cure or respite from this awful debilitating disease. Either way, death is assured.

You see, the door that was her mind, has systematically closed itself off from the rest of her body. It was as if her brain had locked itself in a nuclear shelter whilst awaiting the inevitable end. In essence, slowly but surely, she was shut off from cognitive connectivity to her body.

This is all about Cilla and her eventual relationship with the disease PSP – which is the shortened version for Progressive Supranuclear Palsy.

But before I fully get to the **Me** bit – Cilla's bit – I feel I need to explain a little bit more about PSP.

The description below has been taken directly from the PSP Association's web page – http://www.pspassociation.org.uk/ – and reproduced with their kind permission.

Details of the medical term and associated complications are as follows:

A Brief Guide to PSP

'Progressive supranuclear palsy (PSP) is a Parkinson's-like neurological condition caused by the premature loss of nerve cells in certain parts of the brain. Over time, this leads to difficulties with balance, movement, vision, speech and swallowing.

Research suggests around 4,000 people are living with PSP in the UK at any one time. In its early stages, symptoms can resemble those of other neurological conditions such as Parkinson's, Alzheimer's, stroke or multiple system atrophy; with the result, that initial misdiagnosis is common.

PSP is a very individual condition and symptoms can be experienced with varying degrees of severity and at different stages of progression.

Early symptoms may include loss of balance, falls (often backwards), stiffness and eye problems – this might be difficulty in looking up or down, focusing, double or tunnel vision and dislike of bright lights. Some people can also experience behavioural and cognitive changes including depression and apathy.

PSP is associated with the build-up of a protein called tau in certain areas of the brain. The protein forms into clumps (neurofibrillary tangles), which are believed to damage the nerve cells.

Like many other chronic conditions, there is currently no cure for PSP. However, many of the symptoms can be managed to help you achieve the best possible quality of life.

PSP tends not to run in families and the disease is not currently believed to be inherited. However, research indicates that some people may have a genetic disposition which makes them more susceptible.'

So there you have it.

That is the straightforward definition of PSP and, in basic terms, what it is all about. However, the clinical overview does not take into account the living, breathing, day-to-day, sun worshiping, ice-cream-liking, fun-loving, family-oriented person that was once a PSP sufferer. Nor is it meant to, since it needs to be clinical and straight to the point to make sense.

Nevertheless, there is a personal, human element to this; certainly one that cannot be ignored or described in any other way than through the eyes of those directly involved.

It is one that has a unique story attached, since each and every story about PSP, although similar, is moderately different with one exception: the outcome. How each sufferer copes with it on a day-to-day basis is as much to do with the people around them as it is to do with both the surroundings and the individuals involved.

Before I start, I would like to highlight a little-known fact by conveniently quoting one name. This is to give you some perspective of how sufferers in the early stages of the illness are sometimes perceived. That name is Dudley Moore. Due to no fault of his own, Dudley had a reputation for drinking heavily – even though this was not the case. This myth was spurred on by the success of the film *Arthur*, where he was portrayed as a rich, womanising alcoholic. It is generally an unknown fact that Dudley developed and eventually died of complications caused by PSP.

In essence, the early signs of the illness just added to his unjustified reputation. His frequent stumbling and speech slurring were, initially, put down to alcohol excesses. And no matter how it was explained, the public giggled and collectively agreed that he was playing true to his character's role. To enhance this point, I would like to refer you to www.youtube.com/watch?v=VVWGutY0xbw and beg you to watch it in its entirety.

Alternatively, just type in **Dudley Moore PSP**, and the link will come to you.

You Are Not Alone

There is something else that is equally important for you to understand about PSP: you are not alone. Apart from Parkinson's, PSP sufferers share a common relationship with Corticobasal Degeneration (CBD), and from the following you can see the similarities. Nevertheless, from beyond this point I shall be concentrating on just PSP despite the similarities of the two conditions. However, any future advice can quite easily benefit both conditions and other related illnesses.

Once again the highlighted description has been taken directly from the PSP Association's web page and with their kind permission:

A Brief Guide to Corticobasal Degeneration (CBD)

'Corticobasal degeneration (CBD) is a degenerative brain disease affecting people from the age of 40 onwards. Although there are similarities to PSP, with similar nerve cell damage and the build-up of a protein called tau in certain parts of the brain, the classical clinical picture is quite distinct.

However, people diagnosed with CBD may go on to develop features of PSP and vice versa. Overlap between the two conditions is now well recognised.

Cognitive problems are common in CBD and are often one of the first symptoms that families notice, particularly apathy, impulsive behaviour, changes in empathy and language changes.

Other signs of CBD may include progressive numbness and loss of use of one hand. There may also be jerking of the fingers, slowness and awkwardness and the feeling of having an 'alien limb' – with complex unintentional movements of one limb causing problems with normal motor tasks.

Gradually the arm and/or leg on one side is affected and then the arm and/or leg on the other. People with CBD often have trouble controlling one hand when doing everyday things such as writing or tying shoelaces – tasks that involve individual muscle movements we take for granted. Eye movements can also be disturbed but this is less common than in PSP.

There are currently no treatments for CBD but there are a number of ways to help manage the symptoms and simple practical solutions that can help get around some of the problems people living with CBD experience.

As with PSP, there are no simple tests or brain scans for CBD to help neurologists diagnose the condition. CBD is often initially misdiagnosed as a stroke or Parkinson's disease.'

Me

N ow, let us get to the 'Me' bit.

'Why me?' That was the question Cilla openly asked herself *only once*. Before long she readily accepted the unanswered demand for a response, and towards the middle years of her illness she no longer pondered this, since it seemed to her to be so irrelevant and wasteful. After a brief period of time the question seemed redundant and far less important to her than her dwindling sight, mobility and speech.

Suddenly, she looked back on her life to see how or where it all went wrong... and in truth, there was no one defining piece of evidence pointing her in any direction, or for her to come to any real conclusion. In fact, did anything in her life ever go wrong? Perhaps you, the reader, or sufferer from PSP, can see if there are any similarities in your life compared to hers? Even Cilla did not come to any firm assumptions about her lifestyle or, indeed, about herself. However, what she did know is that she hoped and prayed that others would not succumb to the same life she was then leading... if you can call it life. Despite this thought, she knew that once diagnosed there was nothing that could be done; certainly, nothing in her lifetime. This though was something she would have liked to amend, and later you can see how she did this.

I suppose, by eventually understanding Cilla, you will get to know some of the answers well before she was able to... or at least tried to.

Oh! By the way, names shall be ruthlessly dropped during the writing of this book, and for that, I offer no apology... it is what it is.

I shall now continue by giving you a summary of her life from birth until now, despite how it actually turned out.

During the reading of this book you will find out exactly how agile she used to be – although later in life, back surgery would turn out to be the first thing to reduce her mobility, but certainly not her will!

Cilla was born on Saturday 23rd of July 1949 in a little-known hospital in Lyndhurst named Fenwick, in the beautiful county of Hampshire, England.

Ironically, and in no way connected to this story, this tiny hospital is located within spitting distance of the Waterloo Arms, which sets the opening scene in Shelby Locke's first novel *Stepping*.

Anyhow, located on the edge of the New Forest in Hampshire, she could not have wished for a better start in life. However, at the time, her parents – Joyce and Douglas Upson – lived several miles away in Sylvia Crescent, Testwood, near Totton. This meant that, for Douglas, travelling to the hospital on a regular basis was to be limited.

Since her mother was convinced she was going to have a boy, she was ill-prepared for the eventual birth of a girl, and had not equipped herself with an alternative or relevant name. Urged on by the Nurses and in haste, she took a name from a book she was reading at the time, and Priscilla Jane Upson was immediately named there and then – much to her father's disgust. To make her name more palatable to himself, he, and only he, adapted her written name to Scilla. By doing so, he incorporated the name of one of his favourite flowers, thus reflecting her subsequent delicate beauty.

However, at a birth weight of nine pounds and nine ounces, Cilla – as she became known – initially lived with the nickname Ten Ton Tessie; ironic really, since she spent most of her youth and early twenties looking like a stick, and even earned the tag beanpole!

For her though, she had a whole life ahead of her to look forward to... although just before she died at the tender age of sixty-six, she looked back and felt there was much she had not achieved or experienced. In reality, however, and compared to others, she had been lucky enough to live quite an extraordinary life. And fortunately for us, she was a prolific diarist, and had also been able to recollect some of what you are about to read. Furthermore, I appreciate that some of the experiences you will read about do go outside the ordinary, mainly due to other people's influences – like that of her father. She was also extremely fortunate to meet some very famous people over the years – which she took in her stride. This was made especially easy since that was the environment and times she lived in.

At an early age, and with an older brother and sister in the wings, she should have expected a more comfortable start in life than she actually had, but this did not take into account how much the age difference meant. Paul was fifteen years older than she was, and Angela was ten when she was born, meaning they were slightly too old to be bothered with a younger sister. So by her fourth birthday she was aware that things were not going to go all her own way.

During her early years, her brother Paul spent a few years serving in the army due to conscription, whilst her sister Angela saw her as a bore and a distraction from boys. Although to Angela, having a younger sister did occasionally have its uses... For instance, household chores she was supposed to do herself were conveniently left to Cilla to do! And this was something that must have been a real issue in Cilla's life, since in our early years together this subject came up several times.

Not long after the aforementioned realisation that not all would go her own way, the family upped sticks and moved to Witt Road in the small village of Fair Oak, another idyllic part of Hampshire. This was the first of many moves, since Cilla was soon to find out that her mother had itchy feet – a nomad, if you like.

Incidentally, both Cilla and Paul shared and independently recalled a very happy and memorable occasion in their lives, and one that related to this next move. Just before Paul was due to be demobbed from the army in August 1954, he received a letter from his parents stating that they had recently moved house. The address they had given him meant nothing, as he had never heard of Fair Oak before, and had no idea where it was. He asked his comrades in arms if any of them knew the location... and they all came back with a resounding 'No'. Left to work it out for himself, and in the heat of the day, Paul caught trains and buses alike before ending up near what is now Marwell Zoo. From here, he blindly walked the several remaining miles with a heavy trench coat and full kit bag. As he approached the area he thought was the right locality, he spied a very young blonde girl looking anxiously up the road toward him. She soon appeared to be jumping up and down in excitement at seeing him. Realisation soon dawned on him that this must be his little sister Cilla, and he called out her name – which instigated a reaction in her as she started to run towards him.

From Cilla's perspective, she told me this:

'I was four and vividly remembered being told that my big brother was coming home from the army on a specific day. I felt excited since I had little recollection of him, but just having an older brother was exciting enough. On the day, I anxiously waited and waited at the end of the road for what seemed like hours. My parents gave me their blessing for me to wait and, in truth, there was little fear in those days about anything untoward happening to a four-year-old girl waiting in the quiet streets of this sleepy little village.

Since I was told Paul was not sure where we lived, I felt privileged to be the one to show him. I remember the skies being clear and the weather on that day was generally hot. Eventually I saw a figure approaching in the distance and my excitement caught the better of me. I started to jump up and down when I could finally see the uniform which confirmed it was who I had been waiting for! He called my name, and without a second thought I flew up the road and into his arms. I cannot describe how proud I felt as I walked home hand in hand with my big brother... and he was still in uniform. I kept looking up at him thinking I was the luckiest girl alive.'

When prompted further on the move to a new house, she noted:

'I suppose the biggest difference I noticed after the move was the size of the house compared to the bungalow we had just left. To me, the stairs in the house seemed to go on forever! For the first time in my life, I had to use stairs to get to my bedroom – which was a big deal to me! Like most children, getting up and down stairs was a doddle, but thinking about it now only makes me feel sad. As usual, I would take these stairs at twos and threes at a time, hanging onto the bannister for support and using it to launch myself into the air. Then it was oh, so easy, and without effort. I would land like a coiled spring ready for the next thing to jump. I loved stairs and, at the time, could not ever remember just walking up or down them!'

With new moves came new friends, and since she made them easily she had plenty. Running, jumping, skipping and climbing activities were all matter of fact, and even childhood illnesses were there to overcome and defeat.

It seemed that she barely had time to adjust to that move before there were rumblings of another one on the way. As usual, most of the moves in their lives were instigated by her mother, but she did not always have it her own way. For example, their next move in 1956 was to be one of the greatest thrills of Cilla's life and, to her father, one of the most expensive to date.

Little Timbers (now reverted back to the original title of Hall Lands Cottage) was a smallholding of some three-plus acres and was literally situated just down the road from their present home in Fair Oak. Unusually, the purchase was made less complicated due to the fact that her father somehow knew the woman who owned it. After some simple negotiations and a firm handshake, the deal was done; no initial involvement with solicitors or estate agents, just a common sense agreement. For the princely sum of £2,350 – to be paid off at £10 a month – the family moved into a world of dreams.

Here Cilla could keep animals of all kinds, and was at an age where she wanted to shelter every type of creature known to man; each animal they acquired had a unique tale attached to how the family came to own them.

Tarla, a short-coated Alsatian and already a family pet, was her guardian who would later give birth to at least ten puppies. Mike, the black half-Border Collie and half-Labrador was given to her by her brother's then girlfriend Eve. Thomas, a stray tabby cat, was found in the loading bay of the then famous Edwin Jones Department Store in Southampton where her father worked. Her father once told her that he could not resist sharing his sandwiches with Thomas during his lunch hour, and a special bond was created there and then between the two of them. Apparently, Thomas was a great mouser, and I am sure Edwin Jones suffered a mouse epidemic after her father brought him home. A year later, and on another memorable occasion, she excitedly accompanied her father to collect Tina the goat from somewhere long forgotten. They arrived at a bleak and desolate farm in Douglas's gleaming dark blue Vauxhall Victor. With a gleeful glint in her eye, Cilla often told me of the story of Tina, kindly leaving quite a few perfectly formed 'nuggets' on the back leather seats to show everybody exactly what she thought of it all. In hindsight, I am sure Cilla's father would have preferred to have used an alternative vehicle for both the trip and the occasion... certainly one more suited to the role.

There was also Sally the pig who happened to be won by Cilla's brother Paul at the fair. He successfully caught her, thus claiming her as his own – although this feat was made even more awkward since Sally was deliberately smothered in grease by the organisers. This made it almost impossible for Paul and the other entrants to get a firm grip, but he finally triumphed after an almighty struggle.

Then there was Smokey, her sister Angela's horse, who she was allowed to ride now and again. To be fair, riding him was a slight exaggeration of the truth, since she straddled him and was mostly led around by her sister.

Topping it all, there was also a mix of small animals such as chickens, rabbits, guinea pigs, hamsters, mice and the occasional slowworm.

However, this story would not be complete without the special mention of two other additions to the family. There were two other pets, which Cilla thought she would mention to me separately, since there was an extra special bond between them due to the circumstances behind their discovery.

Firstly, Donna the duck found her way into Cilla's heart and little menagerie purely by accident.

She recalled:

'My dad and I were walking through St James Park, London, when I noticed something rustling in a bush. Not being shy and always seeking adventure, I decided to investigate, only to find a tiny, lost and bewildered duckling! Dad was beside himself and tried to persuade me not pick it up... but I did. We soon found a park keeper and I asked in a rather determined voice if I could keep her. By acknowledging my argument that the duckling would die if left alone, he decided the most sensible thing to do was to say yes. Of course, it had nothing to do with the pathetic look I was giving him at the time! Knowing my resolve, dad soon relented with not too much of a fight. After all, how could he refuse?'

Secondly, and perhaps under more unusual circumstances than Donna is this next story... especially due to the fact that this particular pet appeared to have adopted Cilla.

She told me:

'I was sitting quietly in the garden one day, and from the corner of my eye I noticed some movement. I turned, and to my amazement there was a jackdaw just looking at me, much in a way it would, while trying to evaluate a critical

situation. Without hesitation, I 'asked' him over with a whistle. With even less hesitation, he accepted my invitation and hopped to my side. I was beside myself with excitement and wonder. His head crooked from side to side for a while, and his eyes blinked several times before hopping right onto my knee. He was heavy, but much lighter than I thought he would be. Gently, using one finger, I stroked him on his head and under his chin as his head tilted slightly to accommodate this. By now, I had already decided to name my newfound friend Jackie! During this time, I felt rather special and hoped the moment wouldn't stop, but Mike came bounding over to see what was going on. Jackie flew off and onto a nearby fence post, but never ventured far away after that. After our initial meeting, we became good friends and we would often swap gifts – a worm or grub for a bottle top, or even, as on one occasion, a piece of polished glass, which to me, at the time was like precious jewellery.'

Cilla never mentioned what happened to Jackie after that, or towards the end of her stay at Little Timbers. All I can say is, through Cilla's memory, Jackie is still living on well beyond her years at Little Timbers, as do the rest of her pets.

On a personal note, I had not seen a jackdaw in years until one recent trip to see Cilla at her final resting place. Now, there is a strange thing about this encounter... mainly due to the location. Winchester Road in Southampton is notoriously busy, and must be considered as the most un-friendliest environment to any creature. However, on this particular day, a jackdaw flew straight onto the carriageway and in front of my car. Of course, I braked, but the jackdaw had already taken flight and landed safely on the pavement to my left. I watched it carefully as I slowly passed... and I am certain it watched me as close as I watched it!

Anyways, the menagerie would never be complete, as she still wanted more additions... but to no avail! Her father was adamant that, thanks to Cilla, they had enough creatures to fill a small zoo. Despite his continual protests, she felt assured that if another desperate creature needed homing, then her father would concede and find a little space somewhere.

Feeding the hoard was made much easier by the fact that her mother, by now, was working in the kitchens at Cilla's local junior school. As a result, her father would, at the end of the school day, regularly collect her from class and garner the swill from the kitchens to share out amongst the various animals at home. From what I understand, the animals never went hungry! Although I am not certain what happened during the extended school holidays.

It was here at the smallholding that Cilla first met Gillian Emery – Gillian still lives on the farm – who along with Dilys Owen eventually became close companions and friends. Unknown to many, they would together roam the local wilderness for adventures. She vividly remembers them both climbing atop a horse – named Gypsy – kept at Gillian's father's dairy farm. Once mounted, they occasionally strapped themselves together for support with a waspie belt, which was generally designed to be worn around the midriff to make the waist appear visibly smaller. Given the nature of this narrow-gauged garment, it meant they were securely joined together with very little breathing space. Their logic was flawed, however, since if one of them lost balance, then they both toppled off. When that happened – and it did a lot – they just dusted themselves down and got back on again!

Gillian recalled:

'Cilla, me, my brother Austin, sister Diane, cousins Edward, Morris, John and Christine, along with friend

Janet – who owned Gypsy – decided to 'borrow' Father's four-wheeled trolley which he used to transport cattle feed around the farm. The purpose was to collectively sit on the trolley and cascade down the steep gravel hill from the farm until we reached Mortimers Lane at the bottom. The distance from top to bottom is about a quarter of a mile and the trolley was without brakes. If there was a problem on the way down, we would all bale out and into the bushes. Of course, this would be impossible today because in those days there was hardly any traffic.'

This type of story was typical of Cilla, since Gillian added:

'I was very shy and held back most of the time, but Cilla was always the one to lead us, despite her being at least a year younger. She always came across as being more grown up, daring and adventurous.'

Cilla certainly came across as being fearless and ultimately, nothing seemed to faze them!

Here, on Gillian's father's farm, she learnt what it was like to taste fresh warm milk straight from the cow's udder. Likewise, the girls used to lie down below a black treacle tap and taste the splendour as it seeped out. My ignorance led me to ask... and I now understand that this treacle-like substance – now identified as molasses – was used in the mixing of silage. Whatever its use, they enjoyed the warm syrupy taste that was free and on tap!

At the time, they knew nothing of the hidden dangers on a farm, so blissfully carried on exploring unabated. As any farmer will tell you, a farm is an extremely hazardous place for children to play in. Fortunately, they did so without harm or injuries, despite playing on dangerous machinery, rusting equipment that sometimes featured sharp protruding parts, and in high places above the aforementioned paraphernalia. There were also other dangers to consider which they only seem to highlight in today's society, which include poisoning, disease, drowning and suffocation!

As far as they were concerned, at the end of the day a quick rinse in cold water was all that was required to safeguard themselves from germs; they felt that this was sufficient enough for overall protection. Back then, in days now so remote, the thought of continually washing themselves with a solution that would kill 99.9% of all household or commonly known germs was furthest from their minds!

As shocking as this might sound, it was here that she first experienced smoking. Gillian and Cilla stole some rolling tobacco from Gillian's grandfather's tobacco pouch, which they found lying around in the kitchen. They quickly ran from the house and hid in a nearby shed. Since they had neither experience nor rolling paper, they experimented by inserting the tobacco into a hollowed out weed of sorts before somehow lighting the resulting realistic-looking cigarette. The amount of smoke it produced and the disgusting taste should have put Cilla off from smoking for life... but sadly it did not. I only say sadly, since I am convinced that there was a marginal link between this and some of the health problems she experienced later in life. As far as her enjoyment was concerned, that I cannot be sorry for. Anyhow, at a young and tender age, she developed a liking for smoking, and would eventually smoke real cigarettes from then on. Up to her death, and for the last few years of her life, she smoked on average three a day – this eventuality was vastly reduced from her earlier regime of anything between twenty and sixty a day.

Although poignant, and as conflicting as this might sound, in the latter days I found the three a day she then smoked as soothing, reflective, and knew it was something she always looked forward to. With so few pleasures left in life, I hope you will forgive me by saying that by comparison, this one pleasure was the one she relished the most.

As I have already said, this was also the start of her enormous love for animals. Since then, she could not remember a time when she did not have at least one pet as a houseguest. However, due to the illness, it was not possible to keep animals since there would be nobody to look after them and Cilla at the same time. Her last – a nine-year-old Rottweiler named Ruby – passed not long after being diagnosed in March 2012 with bone cancer of her rear left leg joint.

As previously explained, there was no longer a logical reason to have another pet thereafter, since there was no longer any time to train him or her, or dedicate the time needed. This was mainly due to the amount of time Cilla now needed to devote to herself and dealing with the effects of her own illness. Notwithstanding this, we often had frequent pet visitors who were always made welcome. Take Stimpy as an example. My niece Shirine took a well-earned holiday – which coincided with her mum's (my sister Joan's) own holiday abroad. Stimpy, a French Bulldog, is squat and heavy but highly affectionate, and loved being with people. His visits were a welcome distraction, and Cilla made sure that he was always able to get on to her bed by lowering it to its lowest setting.

Anyhow I digress... In 1959 there was a dramatic announcement made by Cilla's father. This announcement prompted Paul to think about his own future; indeed, he was given little choice since his father had told him that there was not going to be any room for him in the next upcoming event. Given this lack of option, Cilla's brother Paul decided to move on and start a family of his own. Quite recently, he admitted to me that he was quite content to stay within the family home and might not have even considered marriage at that time, but under the existing set of circumstances felt compelled to do something.

Apart from Tarla, Mike and Smokey, they rehoused all of the animals before handing Little Timbers into the safe hands of the new owners.

As Cilla explained:

'Tarla and Mike eventually came with 'us' on yet another exciting period in my life.

The reason I have put emphasis on the word 'us' is because there were about to be several major changes in our lives as a household, since the family was about to split up. You see, for reasons that I as a youngster did not fully understand, Paul never did marry Eve, (who gave Mike, the cross bred puppy to Cilla) since they had split just before dad's announcement. Later, Paul felt it was time for him to leave the household to set up home with Maureen, his new future intended. During this time of unrest, everything seemed to happen so quickly, and now seems a blur due to the suddenness of it all.

Ironically, with absolute horror and sadness, Mike would later die at the paws and teeth of my sister's Alsatian dog Max, son of Tarla! Smokey, on the other hand, was advertised for sale and sold through the classifieds in the Southern Evening Echo.

Angela too had plans, and soon left home for new horizons.

During further discussions with Paul, I later found out that although Angela's options were predetermined, Paul's were not and, in essence, forced upon him.

However, what made this move more exciting was the location: Beaulieu! And no, in this instance, I do not just mean the village of

Beaulieu... I mean the actual Stately Home of Lord Montagu of Beaulieu!'

(Unless otherwise stated, references here relate to Edward Douglas-Scott-Montagu, 3rd Baron Montagu of Beaulieu who sadly died 31st of August 2015, just three months before Cilla. The estate was immediately inherited by his son, Ralph Douglas-Scott-Montagu, 4th Baron Montagu of Beaulieu.)

Excitingly, Cilla's father had accepted a job as superintendent of the newly founded Montagu Motor Museum – the former name of what was later to become the world-famous National Motor Museum at Beaulieu.

His tenure there lasted from 1959 until November 1974, where he finally ended up working in the cash office before his eventual retirement.

Cilla, then aged ten, found herself catapulted into a world of mixed ideals and confused statuses. After all, being ten meant having fun at all odds, outweighing any consequences from either her parents or her father's employer, Lord Montagu.

Cilla's profound knowledge of everything Beaulieu always astounded me, and has continually held me in good stead in the writing of this book.

For instance, Cilla further explained:

'I have learnt a lot since those days, and can tell you that in 1952 the first car placed on display in Palace House was a 1903 De Dion Bouton, which was owned by Lord Montagu's father. Added to this there were the 1899 Daimler, 1901 Sunbeam Mabley, 1905 two-seater Vauxhall, 1906 Lagonda, 1899 Benz and an 1896 Leon Bollée. The smell was heady. At that time, there was not much to see by today's standards. The world famous museum you see today had no bearing on its origins. In 1959, the year my father started, the museum moved from inside Palace House to purpose-built accommodation which consisted of several wooden buildings housing more cars and lots of motorbikes. I also remember there being a Spitfire aeroplane (JMR), and two Pullman cars associated with the Orient Express sited outside the museum's entrance. Anyway, what made this even more exciting was our new 'abode' – which was a flat on the third and top floor of Palace House.'

The point of the location within Palace House, to me, is rather significant to the story I am now going to relate to you.

Excitedly, Cilla then went on to explain to me a particular event – which is how I remember her telling me – and is as follows:

As a ten-year-old girl, Cilla was often asked to run errands – which invariably meant negotiating several staircases and a lot of steps in between. These stairs usually posed no problem to her at all... although one day she did have a particular mishap. In that instance, whilst getting the *Echo* newspaper for her father, she miscalculated the distance between the step she was on and the mat several steps below. This miscalculation meant she eventually tripped and tumbled down all six remaining steps, before ending up in a heap at the bottom. The end result meant she was left with a broken right ankle... and worse: a bruised ego and injured pride!

With plaster up to her knee she felt completely restricted, since she had to, initially, be carried up and down the stairs to their apartment. She hated every moment of the enforced six-week incarceration – which was exactly how she saw it! It was like trying to keep a wild animal caged as she worked on various and cunningly different ways to gain freedom. Well before the time she had her plaster removed, she was doing daring feats due to boredom. Against odds and doctor's orders, she even managed to hobble about the building. And through sheer grit and determination, she eventually reached the roof area of Palace House where she often went for moments of solace. Despite her restricted height, from here she could see some distance away – although the many trees and rising hills drastically limited her overall view. She said she felt safe there due to the fact that she could not be seen, and it did allow her to observe others from afar. Her mother and father were unaware of her little 'adventures'! Indeed, at the end of the day, she could even see her parents walking towards Palace House, which just about gave her enough time to clumsily scramble back indoors; they soon arrived home none the wiser!

However, one day, she did recall being caught sight of by Lord Montagu whilst she overstretched and peered beyond one of the battlements. *'Who's that up there?'* boomed a terse voice from below and slightly out of sight. Cilla once again scrambled back into the flat and awaited the inevitable telling off, but it never came; perplexed by this, and years later, she asked her father why she had not been berated for the offence. He frowned before replying, '*Probably because I never got to hear about it.*'

In truth, Cilla was always regarded as her father's favourite child – which meant she was always granted special treats. Holidays that the family once could not afford were now readily available, and being a favourite also meant doing things with her parents her siblings were unable to do.

Two memorable events linked to her favouritism stuck in her mind as she later explained:

'*Being much too young to understand worldly things was one thing, but to express something I had heard so much when growing up was another. You see, I was lucky enough to be taken on a trip to Germany, and was absolutely amazed by the countrified area in which we were staying. Most of the houses dotted around were wooden chalets and every one of them had duvet-type bedding. I know this because every morning as we walked to the bakery, I noticed the bedding being proudly displayed and hanging over their respective balconies. Everything was crisp, clean and brisk.*

Mostly every door and window in the neighbourhood was left open to let the fresh air breeze through every room in the house.

On this particular day, we were walking back towards our guesthouse and away from the bakery, when father approached and stopped a man I had briefly seen earlier. My father always seemed to raise his voice and change his tone when speaking to foreigners because, I guess, it was his way of being better understood. The German gentleman was then formerly introduced to me, and in my best German accent I shouted "Heil Hitler!", stood to attention, raised my arm, and tried to click my heels. My father was mortified, and started to bluster, but the German gentleman just roared with laughter and told him not to mind. As if that was not enough, I further embarrassed my father when he actually mentioned the gentleman's name: Herr Stanka! To a child of my tender years, I found this to be hilarious. When I think back, this episode must have horrified my father, but he never really told me off or pointed out that what I did was wrong; his looks, on the other hand, spoke volumes.

The second event revolved around a first in my life. This again was to cause acute embarrassment to my father. Up until then, and I suppose this generally included a lot of people of the time, I had not been to a Chinese restaurant. My father teased me relentlessly on that day so, for that reason, he only had himself to blame for what was about to happen. He ordered the meal with aplomb, and I must admit, once tasted, Chinese food appealed to me.

The following day, my father and I were walking through the grounds and bumped into a grand old man of the estate, Captain Henry Widnell, a former agent of the estate. Captain Widnell approached us and lowered himself towards me. "Hello young lady... I understand you went to a posh Chinese restaurant yesterday. Now, can you tell me what you had to eat?" Of course I knew what I'd had, since my father had told me every time I asked him... and believe me, I'd asked him a lot! "I had Who Flung Dung." I replied with confidence. Once again the response I got was not what I had expected. Captain Widnell first looked up at my father, and then back at me, before roaring with laughter. The reaction almost mirrored the response I had had from Herr Stanka at my ignominious faux pas. In this instance, my reply delighted Captain Widnell so much that he often repeated the story to anybody who would listen. At the time, I was convinced I had yet again said something wrong... Of course, my father's little joke on me had backfired on him, but once more he took it all to heart and in good humour.'

On the other hand, Cilla's brother Paul saw things from a different angle, and following her death, he readily told me a story about the subject of favouritism. Of course, there was no malice involved, and looking into his face as he told the story proved he was looking back with only love in his eyes.

The story starts with Paul having a rare bonding moment with his father Douglas.

He explained:

'There was a time in life when I realised my father knew he was not going to be around forever, and surprisingly asked if I would accompany him to London. The trip to London was more significant to my father, since that is where his roots were firmly planted. I saw it as him taking a last trip down memory lane. It was also suggested that I drive, giving father a break as he was not in full health at the time; this in itself was odd, since he rarely let anyone drive his car.

On the way, it was necessary to stop at Fleet for a comfort break. After fifteen to twenty minutes, we returned to the car to find two policemen examining it. As we approached the car, we were asked who the driver was... not the owner, mind you... the driver. Of course, I said I was. To which the reply was that I was going to be prosecuted for having a bald tyre on the car. In due course, it seemed that any argument I put forward fell on deaf ears, and a ticket was duly given – but not until I had changed the tyre.

Once on our way again I remonstrated to father, to which he said, "Well, as the driver, you are responsible for the safety of both the vehicle and passenger." If anything could make the situation any worse, he even made me pay the fine and take the points on my licence! In Cilla's case, he always allowed her to use the car and always turned a blind eye to any little misdemeanour or little accident.'

When Paul shared this anecdote, I do not think he ever felt that the story was anything but laughable; but I am sure it emphasised the very point about Cilla being a favourite.

That aside, not long after they moved into Palace House, her father decided he would like to keep tropical fish. This was to be the start of one of his many hobbies, which already included icing cakes, embroidery, fly-fishing, gardening, photography and Super 8 filming.

 Happily, the latter has given the family many hours of solace over the years, since it has given them the ability to still see loved ones who have now sadly passed... and this now includes Cilla.

And yes, I did say icing cakes and embroidery!

Douglas was one of those people who wanted to experiment with all sorts of pastimes – including the unusual. In those days, it was common for women to be involved in these activities, but he never shied away from any challenge. Cilla remembered, with great fondness, walking into the kitchen and finding her father practicing his icing skills on empty biscuit tins.

Anyhow, back to the story. A large tropical fish tank was duly purchased, and along with the many fish came the necessary paraphernalia: filters, lights, gravel, weeds, miniature stone castles and the right sort of feed arrived in various packages. The tank was eventually installed, and impressive it looked! Vibrant lights shone upon even more vibrant fish of all types, giving Cilla the impression of a deep sea wonderland... until one disastrous day, when tranquillity was turned into mayhem as the tank, for whatever reason, exploded into tiny shards of glass and a plethora of debris which seemed to go everywhere. With fish flapping and gasping all around their feet, they did their best to contain everything and create an emergency environment for the near-to-death and now homeless aquatic residents. To make matters worse, there was a horrific scream from the room below. This was soon followed by an angry tirade coming from none other than Lord Montagu, who unfortunately found himself the regrettable victim of a soaking as water seeped through the ceiling and into his private apartment below! The ensuing clearing up operation involved everybody, including Lord Montagu, who soon took control and oversaw the clean up. Realising the safety of the fish was paramount, and that the situation could not have been foreseen, he soon forgave the Upson family for the unexpected drenching.

All That Jazz

In July 1956 – and as you may have already worked out, well before Cilla's father became involved with Beaulieu – a meeting took place with His Lordship and a group of men from the Yellow Dog Jazz Club, which was then based at the Portswood Hotel in a suburb of Southampton. The men had approached him about holding a future jazz-based event within the estate grounds. Lord Montagu decided that with the sad demise of previous but successful activities, he would accept a fifty-fifty split of the proceeds and thus granted permission.

By the time Cilla and her parents arrived, the Beaulieu Jazz Festival was well established. Here, and over the next few years, Cilla would meet a vast array of famous jazz superstars such as Nat Gonella, Jonny Dankworth, Acker Bilk, Ronnie

Scott, Humphrey Lyttleton, Kenny Ball and George Melly – to name a few.

Coincidentally, following the premature death of Douglas Upson in 1979, Cilla's mother Joyce moved into a warden-controlled block of flats in Gosport. A few years later, Nat Gonella also moved into the self-same block. Surprisingly, they became neighbours, and soon rekindled their friendship, where it did not take them long to find time to reminisce about their moments at Beaulieu. The town of Gosport also recognised Nat Gonella as a local and national celebrity, by later naming a plaza near the Civic Offices in his honour.

Anyhow, by the fourth year of the festival, up to and onwards of five thousand people were attending, thus making this one of the most successful European jazz events of its kind.

What could possibly go wrong?

Beaulieu 1960

W hat had started as a family affair, where cushions had been scattered around the grassed areas for people to sit on and absorb the music, had now become a mammoth event. But from Cilla's point of view, and during this period of time, there was plenty of impishness for a mischievous eleven-year-old to get on with...

Often, from her vantage point on the supposedly out of bounds battlements, Cilla would soak up the atmosphere as the music wafted across the lawns and grounds. Sometimes she would even sneak under the stage, and just as often back stage, where organised chaos was the order of the day. It was here that she met most of the stars of the events. Cilla also got to know many of the characters running the limited side shows that were brought in to support the event. Here, she remembers having a free reign to roam at will – and inevitably appreciated the music which she always enjoyed. At this point, a one-time Victorian galloping horses roundabout had been converted into a makeshift stage, and some of the galloping horses had been removed from the carrousel and used as decorative features. Here, they had been raised higher so they could be seen by the audience towards the back.

Cilla even mentioned on more than one occasion, and with fondness, meeting Cole Mathieson, who owned and ran the famous Concorde Club in Eastleigh. Whether this was related to the event or not I am unsure, but it would not have surprised, me since it was here at Beaulieu that she had first met him. It was certainly a fitting event for his type of expertise and profound love of jazz.

Also, and unknown to her at the time, Cilla later found out that one of the participating audience was none other than Rod Stewart. She was thrilled to eventually find this out, as she later became a huge fan of his. She even romanticised the fact that they could have met briefly during his visit – although in reality there was probably little chance of that actually happening.

Poignantly, plans were afoot shortly before her death to obtain tickets for her to see him at the Ageas Bowl in West End where she lived, and although by then she was almost blind, her love for listening to music never waned.

Anyhow, although now strictly forbidden, Cilla would often mix with the crowds and think nothing of sitting on the edge of the stage – before being caught and moved on by either Lord Montagu, her brother Paul, or one of her parents.

Paul, along with his brother-in-law John were employed as part-time security guards over the weekends. It was their job to make sure there were no stragglers left on the premises at the extreme end of the day. They also had to make sure that people did not hide in the grounds to save money by not paying the following day's entrance fee. What better an instrument to use to flush them out than Max the Alsatian? One method Paul employed was to release Max into the undergrowth and large shrubs, and then watch in amusement as hordes of people rushed out trying to avoid the snarling and snapping jaws of an incensed Alsatian!

Believe it or not, and on a separate occasion, Max and John had cause to chase some of the revellers onto and along the museum roof. This resulted in John eventually crashing through a skylight and, fortunately for him, landing in the rear of one of the cars on display. Although injured with a fracture and small cuts, his wounds were far less than they would have been had he either hit the metalwork of the car or worse still, the floor. Max, however, continued on his way and eventually cleared the interlopers.

So far so good, and all in all, this event pleased the music lovers, jazz aficionados and groups alike.

However, it was in this inauspicious fifth year and over the August Bank Holiday weekend that things started to go wrong. The highly successful Beaulieu Jazz Festival was soon to become infamous – mainly due to the riotous behaviour of a few which eventually spilled over and unceremoniously became known as 'The Battle of Beaulieu'.

That weekend it was estimated that the attendance figures would be around the ten thousand mark – which vastly overshadowed the 1956 audience of some four hundred patrons.

Mindful of recent experiences, and due to the expected numbers, specific procedures had been put into place. Special teams of army personnel from the Irish Guards were intentionally sought to help control the crowds. At five shillings a night, spectators could either stay in their caravans or tents in a specially designated field selected for its proximity, and the chosen Irish Guards were responsible for this and other high-volume areas.

Already there were problems brewing between the now established 'Trad' (traditional jazz lovers) and 'Mod' (lovers of modern jazz) factions. For reasons unknown to anybody but themselves, a group of hooligans decided that Beaulieu would be the venue to settle old scores. It was soon apparent that there was general ill will between the two groups, and had the signs been understood properly, then maybe something could have been done about it – although the actions and determination of some could not have been predicted.

Some, fuelled by alcohol, began to climb the BBC's weight-limited scaffolding which was adjacent to the stage. Others began throwing bottles toward the stage – and it appeared nothing would deter them. Repeated announcements from officials, including Lord Montagu, did nothing but encourage others to join ranks. Clearly outnumbered, the staff were temporarily left helpless, and all they could do was to protect the majority of peaceful music-lovers by moving them to safety. Eventually, gravity, weight and stupidity conspired together and the inevitable happened: the scaffolding collapsed. Incredibly, there were no injuries connected to the collapsing of the scaffolding – despite all the connected electrics, which were live at the time.

Apparently it was a remarkable sight, and to make matters worse, the BBC was actually recording the event live at the time from an adjacent platform. The BBC had, by the end of the day, one camera put out of action, a set of arc lights broken, and five microphones 'lost' or stolen!; either way, they were never seen again!

Cilla also said that she had felt 'miffed' when she heard that somebody had dared to climb up the side of the building and to the roof of Palace House... after all, she saw this area as her very own personal sanctuary.

Amazingly, order was soon restored and the event was allowed to go on. However, and not surprisingly, Lord Montagu was on the verge of cancelling the rest of the event. Thankfully for the majority it was not cancelled, and the remaining days went extremely smoothly.

Incidentally, although I have already said 'the actions and determination of some could not have been predicted', there was precedence on record.

Only three weeks earlier, Saturday the 2nd of July to be precise, a similar and equally famous jazz festival in Newport, Rhode Island, USA experienced a much more serious riot. Here, even the National Guard were deployed due to the disruption. Tear gas and nightsticks were eventually used to quell the mob of more than twelve thousand young men and women. Many of them were fuelled by alcohol. However, the organisers also blamed the content of three recently released films: *Jazz on a Summer's Day*, *A Summer Place* and *Gidget*. These films were released between the years of 1959 and 1960, and are said to have made an impact on the youth of the time. The films were generally little known about here in the United Kingdom, and presumably had no bearing on what happened at Beaulieu.

Beaulieu 1961

On the 13th of March 1961, Cilla's father was given the proud honour of hoisting a blue flag above Palace House. This honour was to publicly announce to all of the villagers, staff and other interested parties that a son and heir to the estate had been born. The current Lord of the Manor, Ralph Douglas-Scott-Montagu, Fourth Baron Montagu of Beaulieu, arrived with a grand fanfare befitting a new and eagerly awaited successor to Lord Montagu. His arrival had been widely anticipated, and the villagers often followed the daily tradition of looking from across the pond to see what, if any, coloured flag would be raised and flown on that day. Lord Montagu could not have been prouder than finally having a son and heir, since he knew the importance of keeping both the estate and traditions going for centuries beyond his occupancy.

Even whilst this was happening, a special administrative panel had been set up to forward plan the next major jazz event. It was understandably thought by the panel that if the Beaulieu Jazz Festival was to further succeed, then certain things needed to change. By restricting the crowds to six thousand, and selling the tickets in advance, controlling the crowds would be much easier. Sensibly, the sale of alcohol was also going to be restricted – despite protestations from a few disgruntled locals.

As it turned out the actual planning paid off, and the festival returned as a resounding success. But there was a snag... one so great that it eventually caused Lord Montagu to close the once highly profitable and well-attended event at Beaulieu for good.

The Beaulieu Jazz Festival panel had, as you know, now introduced a ticketing system to stem the flow and quantity of the attendees. There was also added security procedures put in place to make the whole experience better for everybody. However, there were still many non-ticket holders arriving in the village, which was a great cause for concern – especially for the tenants and villagers. These unwelcome visitors were labelled 'Beatniks', and their intentions appeared to be anything but social. They showed no consideration for the law-abiding villagers and for those attending the ticketed event. Free love was openly expressed in people's gardens, as well as other unsavoury acts which took place throughout the village.

Controlling the event from within was one thing, but to police the whole village and surrounding area was completely another... in fact, impossible! This was going to be a major factor in the final decision.

Cilla said that from within her secure inner sanctum, she could see there was chaos outside, with people everywhere showing no signs of consideration for others. This collective madness, combined with the aforementioned acts of human denigration, was to be the final act which eventually killed off the event.

The event ultimately failed due to outside pressures, and in Lord Montagu's own words to me many years later: *'In its own way, it became too successful... and there are some who do not like others successes...'*

Adventures, Films and More

U p and until then, and despite the negativity, this for Cilla was as exciting as it got... and to be fair for a girl of her age, it was already pretty exciting.

However, situated in an area close to where the National Motor Museum is currently housed, and well away from recent activities I have referred to, was a paddock where Belinda Douglas-Scott-Montagu, Baroness Montagu of Beaulieu, kept her horses.

Due to recent but now bygone days, this interested Cilla a great deal and she soon found herself spending time there talking to the horses. This did not go unnoticed, since Lady Belinda – as she was eventually known to Cilla – soon befriended the little waif.

It quickly became apparent to Lady Belinda that Cilla was keen to learn more about the horses, and in exchange for some grooming and other related tasks, she taught Cilla how to ride and handle horses properly. It was also Cilla's job to clean all the tack and keep it all in good order. The relationship between the two rapidly developed and soon, Cilla had full permission to ride the horses on and within the estate grounds.

There was one particular horse Cilla mentioned quite frequently, and that was Jeanie. Jeanie appeared to be her favourite, since in her diaries she mentioned that it was her ultimate desire to one day own a horse with a similar temperament. Cilla was in her element since this event revived her earlier, but short association with Smokey, her sister's horse.

Cilla's love of horses would eventually extend to her owning her very own horse, Beauty. But more of that later.

Over the ensuing years, Cilla expanded her equine interests and horse riding would soon play a role in another exciting adventure in her life.

The aforementioned adventure I have referred to, began in late 1965 early 1966, and at the impressionable age of sixteen, Cilla found herself among some of the movie 'greats'. Independently of the museums day-to-day routine, much was going on within the grounds of Beaulieu and the associated village of Bucklers Hard. *A Man for All Seasons* was being shot on location there, since the setting was thought to closely resemble the River Thames during the sixteenth century.

Cilla, never one to miss an opportunity, soon got involved, and through Jackie Cummins the wardrobe mistress, began to generally help out. She rapidly found herself heavily occupied in all aspects of fitting, even helping out on makeup. This opportunity may well have come about following a hair care course that Cilla had taken in early 1964.

I never knew what her parents made of her involvement but something I shall refer to later was, I think, quite telling.

Anyhow, in her free time she would socialise with both cast and crew.

She recalled:

'Due to the heat and looking for shade, I once sat down under a tree next to one of the cast. The man turned to me and offered me an extra strong mint – which he appeared to have in abundance, and stored somewhere out of sight beneath the

many layers of clothing he was wearing. I gratefully accepted. We chatted for ages about no particular subject, but I found his low, soothing voice fascinating. After a while, and in the cooling shade of the tree, he explained that his costume was tiresome, heavy and stifling, which was why he was taking a breather under the tree. I offered to help him with his costume, but before much more could be said there was a shout from Mr Fred Zinnermann (The Director)*: "Paul, your presence is required!"'*

Although Cilla had been helping out on costume, she mainly dealt with the many extras on site, not the Stars. So, up until then, she had no idea she was conversing with none other than Paul Scofield (Thomas More).

Soon after that she observed from a distance, and well away from the rest of the cast, the soon to be famous John Hurt (Rich). He appeared to be going over and over his lines whilst fervently pacing up and down. Cilla mentioned with glee that within his isolated bubble, he also appeared to be acting out some of his movements involving his arms, thus giving her the impression of a demented puppet. She also recalls the many takes and retakes Fred Zinnermann made John Hurt do to perfect his onscreen stumble backwards into the mud following a discussion with Leo McKern (Cromwell). As far as Cilla could see, the first take – and first of many – were no different. In her mind, she always questioned why Mr Zinnermann pursued this, and later presumed it was either an in-house joke at John Hurt's expense, or a way of keeping new talent in check. Either way, John Hurt did not seem to be too amused by all the extra attention he was getting because of it.

Another actor she spoke of with affection was Arnold Peters, late of *The Archers* and many cameo roles on TV. Arnie, as he was known to her, shared his lunch with Cilla on two occasions, and dinner on one. She found his gentlemanly demeanour quite charming.

Eventually, and mostly due to Cilla's easy going and laid-back attitude, she met most of the cast and crew, which included Robert Shaw and Susannah York. She was complimentary about them all, but none more so than one particular actor, namely Drewe Henley. Drewe soon swept Cilla off her feet and into a saddle of one of their most spirited horses; these 'chargers' were feisty by comparison to Lady Belinda's much tamer and disciplined horses. Drewe later told Cilla that from what he had observed, she could ride a horse like a man, and was good enough to join him and his colleagues on rides across the New Forest – which they did regularly; however, they only did this with the consent of Fredrick 'Nosher' Powell who was the on-set stunt coordinator and actor. Nosher Powell also agreed with Drewe about Cilla's expertise in the saddle.

In truth, Cilla later confessed to me that she was petrified at some of the speeds they were reaching! Conversely, she was far too scared to fall off, but it appeared nobody noticed, and her actual terror was seen as fearlessness!

There developed in Cilla's words, 'a romance' between her and Drewe, and she always considered this early love encounter and their brief relationship as somewhat special. This, of course, could not last forever and, more importantly, did not go unnoticed by her father!

As the film and its accompanying circus packed up to locate somewhere else, Cilla was made an offer she thought she could not refuse. Apparently, recommended by both Susannah York and Robert Shaw, and a few of the stunt crew including Nosher Powell, Cilla was asked if she would like to go to Spain in the near future to work on the set of *Battle of Britain*.

Cilla's parents – her father in particular – already had reservations about her exploits, and the point I made earlier when I used the small phrase 'quite telling' thus came into play.

As far as Cilla was concerned, this newfound opportunity was far too good to be missed – although being so young, Cilla needed her parents' permission. In those days, there was very little somebody of her age could do about the situation, especially as she needed her parents' permission to get the necessary passport needed to travel abroad, and despite having already been abroad on several occasions, she had always travelled on a supporting parent's passport.

Her news came as a shock to her parents, where discussions were apparently one-sided... and her request was unceremoniously refused out of hand.

Obviously Cilla was devastated by this, but she understood her parents' concerns and soon, albeit begrudgingly, put this chapter in her life behind her. This did not, however, stop her from reminiscing about the 'what if' moment that had sadly slipped through her fingers. I could see the sense of sorrow by the way she stared into the distance when relating the stories of these days gone by. I could also clearly see there was a certain amount of regret and associated disappointment there... and in my eyes she had every right to feel that way.

Incidentally, in 1968 Drewe Henley married Felicity Kendal and later had a son together; sadly, they divorced in 1979 soon after he was diagnosed with manic depression.

I remember one day hearing a squeal of delight coming from Cilla as she watched television. She had been caught rather off-guard, and was beside herself at seeing Drewe when he appeared as Red X-Wing Squadron Leader, Garven Dreis in *Star Wars Episode IV: A New Hope* on video. We later found out that, for some unknown reason, in this film he was mistakenly credited as Drewe *Hemley*. I remember Cilla fast-forwarding to the credits at the end to confirm what she had just seen was real, and was rather disappointed when she saw that his name had been misspelt.

There were more stars for her to meet in the ensuing years, and I took pleasure in listening to her when she reminisced about those heady days in her life. Stars of stage, screen and music had a habit of popping up at Beaulieu, and on many occasions, Cilla would be there to lend a helping hand. She recalled all of these encounters with great affection, and always used to speak highly of those she met.

By 1960, the family had left the Palace House flat and moved a few hundred yards up the road to a tied cottage – which was still in the grounds of Beaulieu and within the shadow of Palace House. Old Gardens, as they were named, were ideally suited and less restricted as far as Cilla's parents were concerned.

During my research, I noted from a diary that the private telephone number at their new abode was Beaulieu 353. Although not significant to the story, it amused me to see such a short number compared to the average eleven digits used today.

Here Douglas purchased one of the very first BMC Minis to be seen on the roads, and with it was delivered, coincidently, the registration number MMM 660: I say coincidently, because working at the Montagu Motor Museum gave the plate more credence when he was seen out on the manor, where the light blue vehicle was often mistaken as a Beaulieu staff car.

Although it would not be allowed now, Tarla the Alsatian would often be seen sitting in the boot with the lid down; a few blankets would sometimes be strategically placed to make the ride more comfortable for her. In those days, it seemed almost acceptable for this sort of thing to happen, especially on short trips out. Indeed, Constable Parker I believe it was, had spoken to Douglas on several occasions about this... sometimes over a cup of tea whilst watching football on the television at the Upson's residence.

The move itself did not appear to concern Cilla too much because she still had plenty to keep herself occupied, and still had access to Palace House and the roof. Indeed, she even had neighbours who also had a daughter of a similar age, and like friends of old, Cilla soon discovered that this newfound friendship quickly developed into a successful pairing. Notwithstanding this move, Cilla still met famous people, almost on a daily basis.

Mr Pastry was a well-known children's entertainer, and well-loved for his slapstick entertaining on both stage and screen. In this instance, Cilla met him at the Gaumont Theatre – now known as the Mayflower Theatre in Commercial Road, Southampton, which will come up again towards the end of the book – where he was appearing on stage. At the end of the performance, a few selected adults and their respective children were invited onto the stage, and I believe that Cilla was less than impressed when her father dragged her forward and onto the hallowed boards. She met Mr Pastry for a second time when he came to visit Beaulieu whilst taking part in a photo-shoot for an advert. I believe the advertisement in question was for BP Super Plus, a petrol formulation.

By now, and on an almost day-to-day basis, Cilla had become used to seeing camera crews, photographers, actors and actresses among others within the grounds. To name just three further examples of people she met: Eamonn Andrews, Honor Blackman and Laurence Harvey.

Apart from the previously mentioned stars, Dame Margaret Rutherford always stuck in Cilla's mind. Although I am uncertain of Cilla's age at the time, there appeared to be a special bond struck up between them. 'Miss Rutherford' – as Cilla addressed her when talking to me – would often tell countless tales. It appeared that in her capacity as an actress, she seemed quite enthusiastic about all the subjects they ever discussed. 'Outrageously flamboyant' were the words Cilla often used to describe her. However, there were times during their discussions where Miss Rutherford would suddenly stop talking because she had lost her thread... but this never deterred the two of them from quickly picking up on another subject and carrying on as if nothing had happened.

In 1964, Cilla was formerly introduced to Diana Dors. Being at that 'impressionable age' as her father would say, she instantly fell in love with the star that Diana Dors was. Seeing Diana Dors reinforced Cilla's belief that smoking was cool. The associated glamour and personality of the person Diana was, impressed Cilla greatly, and more surprisingly, overrode everybody else she had already met.

I am also convinced that Cilla's eventual love of everything Marilyn Monroe was connected to this particular meeting.

Cilla finally met Diana again in February 1968 at a Beaulieu dinner dance held in the Domus.

Beaulieu would never really leave Cilla – as you will find out later – and even though she eventually moved away from Beaulieu, on a flying visit to see her father one day in 1973, and accompanied by family, she called into the museum and was fleetingly introduced to the then current teenage heartthrob David Cassidy.

Some of the estate staff, for instance Captain Widnell who has already been mentioned, are classic examples of interesting personalities found within Beaulieu. In fact, some of these were just as fascinating to Cilla as many of the already named and notably world-renowned visitors.

Then there was Graham Walker, the famous and successful motorcyclist, broadcaster, journalist and, incidentally, father to an equally famous Murray Walker. Although Cilla had less to do with him, she had met him on many occasions. Graham was mainly responsible for the motorcycle section of the museum, and a great advocate of two-wheeled transport.

Take Michael Sedgwick as another example. As curator of the then newly named Montagu Motor Museum and motoring author, he was a fascinating character in his own right, but a story he told Cilla had a profound effect on her.

Whether for effect or not he had the ability to capture one's imagination, and on this particular day he told Cilla this story, which, in her words, went as follows:

'Michael told me he was sitting in the front room of one of the houses situated near ours in the Old Gardens. It was a particularly hot day and the French doors were open to let some air in to circulate. As he was sipping tea, he could hear many feet approaching the house from within the

garden. This was unusual since he could also, and distinctly, hear the sound of gravel being trampled on outside the French doors. Michael knew this could not be the case, because outside the doors was a lawn... the gravel courtyard had been laid to lawn many, many years before. To make this story even eerier, he said he could also hear the Gregorian-style chanting of monks. What made this story so remarkable was the fact that this happened in broad daylight, not as one would imagine at the stroke of midnight.'

Cilla's interpretation was that this was a ghostly manifestation of some of the many monks who lived and prayed on the site. Perhaps, in their day, their regular daily route took them through the garden setting... who knows?

I once raised this subject with Derek Maidment, the keeper of exhibits, who told me there were many such stories. Indeed, he added his own spin, and told me of a legion of Roman soldiers passing through the houses before disappearing through a solid back wall.

Cilla also told me that she often felt a presence in the cottage they lived in, in the Old Garden block. She distinctly remembered sudden changes in temperature for no apparent or particular reason at all. Sometimes intense heat would suddenly be replaced by a cold so defined you could see the breath vapours coming from your own mouth. I mention this, because the cottages were not modernised at that time, and they certainly did not have small luxuries like central heating.

In 1966, Cilla's parents eventually realised that they could not stay in a tied house forever, and began to look elsewhere to live. Some fifteen years after moving to Beaulieu, they soon found that there were significant changes to owning a house and most notable of these were the prices.

However, it was not long before they relocated to a nearby property: being just three-and-a-half miles away and reachable within seven minutes, number 11 Arnewood Avenue in Dibden Purlieu was an ideal location for Douglas.

This move did not, however, affect Cilla's treasured and countless memories and so many additional moments during her time as a youth at Beaulieu.

Coincidently, I recently came by an unusual 'curio' still held in Cilla's possession. This 'curio', consists of a single piece of A4 paper and contains a complete set of Cilla's fingerprints! The C.3.-15 form was used to eliminate Cilla's prints from a robbery that took place after the move away from Beaulieu. Cilla recalled the event, and told me that a cabinet had been broken into and several model cars had been taken, although, I now believe this was just one. I am not sure how selective the robbery was, but Cilla was formerly responsible for cleaning both the cabinet and the cars within, hence the need to eliminate her legitimate prints from their enquiries. Cilla was also responsible for cleaning a few of the rare and outrageously valuable 'Lalique' mascots, which were 'housed' next to the display cabinets in question.

Douglas remained involved with Beaulieu until the 29th November 1974, when he eventually retired. Sadly, Douglas only had a few years to enjoy retirement, and suddenly passed away aged sixty-nine on 22nd of March 1979. In relation to this, I recently found a handwritten letter from Lord Montagu sending his condolences to Cilla's mother. In it, he expressed his deepest respects, and said he could not attend the funeral since, at the time of Douglas's death, he was away in India.

Before I move on, I would like to mention that Douglas played the piano as well as the three and four manual pipe organs. Furthermore, he did as he put it, 'a stint' as organist and choirmaster at the Beaulieu Parish Church where he played at Cilla's baptism. That, to my knowledge, was the only religious connection I can find where Cilla was concerned.

Education 1954-1966

It would be remiss of me if I did not mention Cilla's academic career, which I have only briefly touched on when talking about Fair Oak earlier.

The few conversations I had with Cilla about her time at school did not give me the impression that her moments spent there were spectacular. However, she told me she was a hardworking and willing pupil, but later lacked a certain commitment that was required for her to achieve her full potential. She also told me that her education in the latter years was hampered because she was too easily distracted, and casually put this down to her newfound fascination with boys.

I have already mentioned her early connection to Fair Oak, which was later disrupted by the move to Beaulieu, but by all accounts, Cilla loved her time at both Fair Oak Infants and Junior School and Beaulieu Junior School.

Fortunately, Cilla's parents kept most of her reports, which latterly bore out her remarks about her propensity to distractions. Due to her parents' diligence, I have been able to sort through her reports and they are quite telling. Her first report gives her age as five years and five months old. There were twenty-five pupils in her class and she attained a marks score of ninety-five out of 100. This gave her a first in her class, and the teacher had written the following: '*Priscilla has made a very good start, and takes all her work in her stride. She is always cheerful and well mannered.*' Three months later and her scores had slipped slightly, but the class size had increased – although this report reflects the first in its account: '*A very quick child with reading and numbers. I am sure Priscilla will make rapid progress next term. Very good behaviour.*' I also noticed one more remarkable feature about this report, and might as well explain further. The average age group in her class was six years and seven months. This became the norm in her schooling as she always ended up being up to a year younger than most of her classmates. The age difference might also explain why she mentally matured faster than anticipated due to the one-year gap. Physically though, she remained thin, and somewhat under developed.

Her final year in Fair Oak saw her at the age of eight and in a class of thirty-nine. Here she was once more first in her class at just two points off perfect. The final remarks from her teacher were: *'Priscilla has really tried hard all through the term. The exam results are pleasing. Well done, Priscilla, good success in your new school.'* This was signed by her favourite of all the teachers she ever mentioned: Mrs E Treasure.

Somehow, and I could be wrong here, I vaguely remember Cilla saying that Mrs Treasure died in a plane crash. I tried to research this point, but found little evidence to substantiate her remarks to me.

From here Cilla went to Beaulieu, where I was only able to find just one report. The report, dated June 1960, had no formal structure and is simply laid out on a piece of graph paper. Here she attained marks of excellence and ended up third in her class.

Incidentally, only a year or so before she passed away, a group of her former and present carers took her on a round-trip of her childhood haunts, which ultimately led them to Beaulieu. It was here, just outside the school entrance, that the girls stopped the car and allowed Cilla a moment or two to reminisce. This unexpected excursion thrilled her and lifted her spirits to the highest level I had seen for a long time.

From Beaulieu, Cilla attended Priestlands Secondary Modern in the village of Brockenhurst, some six miles away from Beaulieu. Here she started to struggle, and in her first report, dated Autumn 1960, classified her as twenty-seventh out of thirty-three. What is more telling is what is written in her second and final report at Priestlands: Summer 1961 shows that she missed thirty-four days out of 130 in the term. There was also a notable remark from one of the teachers: *'Only fair. Needs to pay more attention.'*

From this and beyond, I sensed that Cilla's parents wanted more from her and started to look around at an alternative school where, they hoped, she would get back on track. However, living in the remote village of Beaulieu had its limitations when it came to higher education. Of course, there were options in the surrounding villages of Hythe,

Fawley and Lymington, but it was obvious that Douglas wanted her to be privately educated.

Despite being baptised, religion never played a big part in Cilla's life, so it was a surprise that she eventually ended up at La Sainte Union (LSU) in Southampton.

I am convinced that Douglas saw the Catholic teaching methods as being the most disciplined. Whether he thought Cilla needed the discipline or not, I am unsure, but he certainly had an agenda where her education was concerned.

La Sainte Union (LSU) was owned and run by the La Sainte Union des Sacrés Coeurs order of nuns, and this Catholic background was generally reflected in the student makeup.

Although he always wanted the best for his little girl, this move was going to cost him dear! I found two receipts for the terms December 1962 and Easter 1963, each made out for the grand sum of £34 and 13d (pre decimal pennies); at the time, the average living wage, based on a forty-five-hour working week, was between £12 to £14.

In all, I am not a hundred percent sure this was a good move on his part, but he was hoping for the best from his daughter in return. Certainly, if he was wanting a good return on his money, then the first report might have come as a bit of a setback. With quotes like, *'Very disappointing'* and *'Priscilla misses some lessons'*, I am sure these comments would not have gone down too well! To be fair though, the overall report was fairly good, so perhaps she could be forgiven a lapse or two. However, her following report threw up all sorts of negative remarks: *'Good.'*; *'Exam results disappointing.'*; *'Priscilla is capable of good work but does not always give of her best.'*; *'More care and concentration needed.'*. And finally, the Reverend Mother, Sister Mary Hilary's summary: *'Priscilla must not be satisfied by her present standard of work, but strive to improve it.'*

The final report from La Sainte Union (LSU) underlines her lack of commitment, and all the tutors underlined similar conclusions. They all agreed that Cilla had the ability, but did not appear to want to apply it. A section in Reverend Mother's summary, dated July 1964, highlights this very point, *'Priscilla should have achieved a better standard than this...'*

Despite this, Cilla often recalled the names of the nuns with affection, but none more so than the Reverend Mother, Sister Mary Hilary. I think this fondness was mutual, and to give you an example of Cilla's impact on the Reverend Mother, Cilla recalled her last assembly where she was unexpectedly singled out.

Incidentally, when speaking of the Reverend Mother, Cilla always allowed herself a bit of theatrics and put on a pretentious voice.

Here she quotes the Reverend Mother as saying this: *'Priscilla, when you first arrived here, we were known as a school for young lady's. However, since your arrival we have become known as a school for gals.'*

I can honestly picture this occasion and can almost hear the words leaving Reverend Mother lips!

Something else Douglas had not taken into account when he made his decision on placement was the logistics of getting Cilla to Southampton on a daily basis. To achieve her schedule, she had to be at the Hythe Ferry Terminal well within departure time, no matter what. However, weather would quite often play a hand in this, since cancellations and delays were not uncommon. Sometimes – and without the means of mobile phones in those days – Cilla would somehow contact her extremely busy father and he would have to drop everything, before setting off on the extremely long journey to Southampton to either drop her off or to collect her. On the outward journey, buses were an option, but these were limited and would often arrive in Southampton far too late for Cilla to attend some of the earlier classes. Of course, from Cilla's point of view, there was also an alternative – which was for her to 'bunk off' altogether and visit one of the many coffee houses in Southampton! Strangely, and unlike Priestlands Secondary Modern, her many absences seemed to go unnoticed, or if they were noticed then they remained unmentioned. I always joked that the school probably felt it performed better without her being there. Ironically, the school only notified Cilla's parents about her nonattendance on one occasion, and oddly, that was when she was off through genuine sickness.

During and between the latter part of 1964 and until mid-1965, Cilla enrolled at the Southampton Technical College in St Marys Street, Southampton. Here, she actually gained a high mark... but unfortunately, there were no supporting comments in the final column of her report to distinguish anything other than a grade of 122 out of 140.

In the Summer of 1965, her formal education came to an end. Yet in early 1966, Cilla's father, still wanting the best for his daughter, enrolled her into a special course in the hopes she would graduate with a diploma.

When I found the documentation concerned, I was slightly confused since I had never heard of a comptometer. Anyhow, a comptometer is an adding machine, which can calculate extremely large sets of numbers.

The course was run by Sumlock Comptometer Ltd, which was situated at 12 Bargate in Southampton, and the documentation I found revealed that: *'Priscilla found the work difficult at times, but by persevering overcame this and passed her Diploma examination at the first attempt, a well-deserved achievement.'*

Correspondence was signed by (Miss) D E Dene, Southampton College Principal.

I do know that Cilla rarely used these skills, but briefly worked in an accounts office just up the road from where she attained her diploma.

Work

N ow, and before she left Beaulieu at the age of seventeen, Cilla was working part-time before finally ending up at Gardner & Young Ltd (from late December 1967 to December 1969).

The part-time employment previously mentioned revolved around bar work, which sometimes included some silver service waitressing. She told me two stories relating to her abilities, or lack of, around the table in this capacity.

Firstly, she recalled:

'I had about two lessons, which were spur of the moment affairs. Handling a spoon and fork together like chopsticks did not suit me well. Then I was thrown in the deep end, as they had a large high-end business bash to deal with and were

short-staffed. I was doing quite well until it came to serving the peas! For some reason, I could not keep the little buggers on the spoon, and leant over to serve the groups boss. As expected, the inevitable happened and I dropped a large spoonful of peas into his beer. The table went silent as I tried to scoop them out with the serving spoon. Goodness knows where I thought I was going to put them and for some reason I placed them on his plate... beer and all! Perhaps sympathy played its part, but I got away with it as he winked at me, lifted his pint with a few peas still swilling around and said "Cheers!" The rest of the table shouted their approval, and joviality took over from what was, until then, a rather dull event.'

No sooner had the dinner been devoured, came the second incident:

'Then it came to the pudding. Once again, I started at the head of the table and asked the boss what he wanted from the cart. He scanned the puddings before choosing the apple pie and custard. As I was serving it, I inadvertently destroyed the pastry top – which turned out to be fortuitous as I spotted a huge area of mould on the apple – so I played it rather cool and completely wrecked the pie before saying that it was off the

menu and returned it to the kitchen. I think he either saw what I had seen, or understood that there was a problem with it. His kindness helped me through the evening and, to top it all, he gave me a hefty tip!'

Now with Beaulieu left behind her, and with significant new things in her life we move on.

At Gardner & Young Ltd, Cilla initially worked in the accounts as a junior clerk, which was only made possible by her father's forward-thinking. Here though, her duties did not require the use of such a complicated adding machine that she had been trained to use, but a smaller run-of-the-mill paper-fed contraption. However, and for some unknown reason, Cilla eventually became their full-time telephonist, in which she soon excelled.

After two years, Cilla moved to Oakley & Watling (from January 1970 to December 1971). Both of these were situated just up the road from number 12 Bargate. Here, having three telephone lines meant she was in constant demand. Nevertheless, one of the perks of the job was the necessity to get cheques signed on behalf of the accounts department. How is this a 'perk' I hear you ask? The company had what they called, 'The Annex' – which turned out to be The Red Lion Pub next door. This late 15th to early 16th Century Grade II listed pub in Southampton's High Street was where the directors and management conducted much of their business. Every Friday, Mr Spalding, the branch director, always insisted that Cilla join him and his associates in a drink or two... or three... whilst she waited for the cheques to be signed.

Who was answering the telephones in her absence is unknown to me.

Incidentally, back in 1912 all the meals that were prepared on board *Titanic* were done so by using fruit and vegetables that came from Oakley and Watling. As an enterprise, Oakley and Watling provided the *Titanic* with all the fresh fruit it required for the trip, which included 36,000 apples, 16,000 lemons and 13,000 grapefruits.

Although I do not have the exact dates at hand, I do know that Cilla worked as a receptionist at Raymond's Hair Salon prior to working at ISR – her next big career move. During this period, there was an incident that shook Cilla to the core, and when she told me about it, I could see that it had initially affected her.

Over a period of a week or so, Cilla left work and walked from the bottom end of town and towards her bus stop further into the city. This was her usual daily route and she kept to it without diversion. It was during this particular week as she was walking this route that she became aware of a man following her. He wore distinctive camouflage fatigues, and gave both the impression and appearance of a soldier. If she stopped, slowed, or turned to look back, he would dart into a nearby doorway or turn around. Although the man's intentions were unclear, the manner in which he was shadowing her felt threatening.

With so few people around at the time, this really spooked her and she became so concerned that she told her father. It was then that the police became involved, who in response devised a plan to use Cilla as bait. Obviously, she was not pleased to be placed in this position, but was told that unless he actually made threatening advances toward her, then there was little they could do. As each day developed so did his boldness, and as he became braver so he ventured closer... according to Cilla, sometimes uncomfortably too close!

It was eventually arranged for Cilla to be watched in such a manner that the stalker would be unaware of a police presence. It was also confirmed by the police that the situation needed their full attention, especially since Cilla now felt she could take no more and was almost in total meltdown over the situation. One day soon after, a Friday I think, she was told to act naturally and take her usual route and try not to do anything that would make him suspicious of the situation. I know this must have been extremely hard for her to do, but in true spirit, she did as requested.

At first, there was no sign of him, but as she ventured further up the street, he appeared from a shop doorway.

At no time did she see anything out of the ordinary, apart from her stalker, who was now far too close for comfort. The situation made her feel extremely vulnerable, because even she could not see any police presence and the street was eerily empty and quiet. By not seeing any evidence of support, she became somewhat agitated and slightly angry.

It was not long before he made his move... which was unfortunate for him on two counts. Cilla's fear then turned to rage, and much to his surprise, she lashed out and started to attack him out of frustration. It took two police officers to get her off him as several others pinned him down!

It transpired that the man was carrying a Bowie-style knife and was eventually sectioned for this and other offences. Apart from this, I know no more than that Cilla was not the first to report his antics, which is why the police eventually showed concern.

Towards the end of the story her attitude changed, and was typical of her enduring spirit. Her parting comment to him was: *'If you are going to stalk somebody in a city, don't wear camouflage! It looks suspicious.'*

In early 1972, Cilla was employed at ISR (International Synthetic Rubber) in Hythe as a receptionist.

Due to Cilla's former star-studded lifestyle, she had developed an approachable manner and nothing seemed to faze her, so on that basis alone being a receptionist suited her. Her position, and working in an area considered by some as the hub of all activity, made the pairing well matched. The reception, in essence, was a meeting place and more importantly, a place to hear the latest gossip. As all Cilla's friends and family can tell you, she remained faithful and loyal to the end. Therefore, once told a secret, she would never divulge its content, and providing the secrecy card was never played, the reception was where everybody congregated to exchange current goings on.

Being the centre of attention did not faze Cilla one bit; indeed, she tended to absorb the attention and effortlessly put others at ease in any given situation, and due to her position within the company and despite occasional strike action, she always tried her best to be on time.

One particular day would be different though, as Cilla relayed:

'I was driving my Mini to work one day and approached the gates where I was confronted by a group of workers that I knew well. Unbeknownst to me, they had called a lightning strike and the guys on the picket instantly recognised the car. They flagged me down and stopped me from entering the plant. They quickly explained that I was not going to enter, and to prove their point, they gathered around the car before collectively lifting it off the ground and physically turning it around. I had no choice but to drive home, take the day off, and explain to my boss later. These were not aggressive men, but the self-same who I would normally drink with in the canteen and in the onsite club on a daily basis.

Despite this, everything then seemed so much more relaxed and manageable. There was no animosity over their actions, and certainly no recriminations. *It wasn't long before they went back to work and I would see them all in the canteen where they were the first to buy me a drink.'*

Cilla also recalled another exciting, if not more dangerous incident whilst working at ISR, as she explained:

'The first I knew about the fire was when the switchboard lights all lit up at once. Then I heard a blast, which sounded remarkably close... a bit too close! I had to follow procedure and obeyed the rulebook as closely as I could. Soon after I heard the blast, one of the onsite firemen ran into the reception and told me to call 999 since the fire was out of hand. By now, I had called all departments to evacuate the area but was told to stay and man my station since the continued need of communication was required. I was not too happy about this, since I knew that we dealt with extremely volatile chemicals onsite. What did make my day was the amount of gorgeous firemen I was soon surrounded by!

I was eventually given the all clear, but no sooner than that had been given there was a further explosion, and all hell let loose as the remaining firemen had to quickly put their protective gear back on. Eventually, I was allowed to leave and the plant was temporarily closed down on safety reasons.'

It was here, during her leisure time, she learned how to play squash – a sport she appeared to excel in. Frequently challenged by the men to play a round or two, she would often win resoundingly. Perhaps this was because she never really took the challenges too seriously, but with bruised egos, the men always demanded a rematch over drinks afterwards.

On the down side, money always seemed to be a problem while working there, since it appeared her wages would not cover her daily expenses. As a result, on Thursday 25th January 1973, she found a part-time job behind the bar at The Malt and Hops in Hythe. For the grand sum of £1.20 an hour plus tips, she felt relieved at receiving some extra income. By all accounts, her time at The Malt and Hops turned out to be more sociable than she expected. It appears that takings started going up soon after her arrival, since her boyfriends, old and new, came to give her added moral support. Many of her socialite girlfriends also dropped the 'in places' in favour of spending time with their good friend Cilla.

In her diary of the year, she also mentioned that her boyfriend of one year, David, a regular at the pub, had just bought a brand new MGB GT! Apart from this, there was definitely romance in the air where David was concerned, but fortunately for me, their relationship eventually waned. Strangely, as I read through Cilla's diary of that year, their passion seemed to turn sour during a well-planned and highly anticipated holiday in Thassos. It would appear that for Cilla boredom set in, and doubts spread due to David's sombre moods. Spending too much time together seemed to be a sticking point as far as Cilla was concerned.

Just before their eventual split, Cilla left her part-time job at The Malt and Hops, which inevitably meant she needed to find another part-time job.

Enter Godfrey Davis Car Hire!

Here, Cilla collaborated with a few of her work colleagues from ISR, one of which was Nigel Pope.

Nigel remembers the partnership well, and insists it was more fun than work, especially as Cilla was the only female in the group. Their job was to pick up returned hire cars from the car park at the rear of the then Post House Hotel (formerly the Skyways Hotel and now the Holiday Inn) just outside dock gate eight in Southampton. From there, they would take the cars to various locations, mostly south of Birmingham. Their only drawback was that a Godfrey Davis employee was always there to keep an eye on things... and for good reason.

The Godfrey Davis employee drove a minibus, which was there to bring them all back from their ultimate destination. Invariably, the final destination was Neasden in North London – although at the time other destinations were just as possible and, by all accounts, just as dreary. In most instances, they did not know what cars they would be driving, and would always jostle for the best vehicle.

On one occasion, Cilla spied a brand new top of the range Ford Capri in the car park. Fast-thinking, she raced ahead of her colleagues, who were unexpectedly caught in her wake and enviously watched as she 'bagged' the keys to the Capri. Finally, after the rest of the cars were allocated, the convey set off and headed for the motorway. Once they reached the M3, the cars set off at pace, leaving the beleaguered Godfrey Davis employee way behind. The road before them soon became a racetrack as traffic was light and they were not paying for the petrol. It did not take Cilla long to gain an advantage as her powerful car pulled further and further ahead. Soon she was out of sight of the others, and as the road opened out she thought she would see how fast she could take it. With the radio blaring, she soon became disturbed by a strange noise. Nothing she did would stop the noise, and then she realised the sound was coming from behind... and the blue flashing lights she could now see were associated with the noise.

The two police officers by the roadside appeared, to the gaggle of car drivers in the ensuing Godfrey Davis convoy as they passed, to be in intense conversation with Cilla. In London, and at their final designated point, the drivers anxiously awaited Cilla's arrival. Convinced she had been given a ticket for speeding, they all jeered as she leapt out of the car. Characteristically she was grinning from ear to ear, and briefly bowed before them whilst stating that she only received a verbal caution for the offence. Much to her colleagues' disbelief, Cilla told the police that she had not noticed doing the speeds they said she was going, and added that had she known the car had that sort of capability, then she would not have chosen it. Nigel is convinced to this very day that if any of the other drivers had been caught doing the same speeds, then they would definitely have been given a ticket for speeding.

On a second occasion, Cilla and another driver went missing for over an hour, leaving the remaining concerned group to consider their next move. All of a sudden they both arrived. The Godfrey Davis employee was furious since this had set him back by a considerable amount of time, and getting back to Southampton would now leave his strict schedule tight. Some of the awaiting drivers had suspected, for no good reason, naughtiness had taken place and muttered among themselves before expressing their collective disapproval. Eventually, the other driver accompanying Cilla felt compelled to explain that she had run out of petrol and he had stopped to help. *'Honest!'*, he exclaimed, as he naïvely held his hands up in the air and stretched them towards the others. *'Here, you can smell my hands if you don't believe me. . .'* As soon as he had finished his sentence, he realised the full implications of his words and gestures. *'No! No! Petrol! Petrol!'* he shouted... but it was far too late. Even the seriously straight-laced Godfrey Davis employee fell about laughing. Cilla's face reddened at the innuendo and was frequently reminded of the story for many years to come.

Cilla's diaries revealed that she had a love-hate relationship with her employers at ISR – although she tried to make the best of her time there and as interesting as possible.

Once again, Nigel recalls one of the escapades they got up to:

'As you know, Cilla was the receptionist/telephonist at ISR, located in the administration building. During the working day most people would pass through, always engaging Cilla in chat so she would get most of the gossip. She also had to use the Tannoy to call people in the plant. It was one of my regular aims to distract her whilst she was making these calls so she would break down in a fit of the giggles.

A particularly moody and gruff shift manager would often pass through reception when he was on days. His aim was to go through reception and to the office of the works director. On passing Cilla, he would frequently stop for a chat and even buy her a coffee from the vending machine situated within sight of Cilla's desk. This was, in itself, quite surprising, since he was particularly mean with his money.

One day, we decided to wind him up by jamming the cups in the machine so that when it vended coffee it would pour straight through with no cup in sight. This wound him up, not because of the loss of coffee, but because he had lost his precious money in the process. It did not take him long to assess what was going on and to counteract our actions – and he began to bring in his own supply of plastic cups. This meant that if no cup appeared during the vending process, then he would open the little Perspex door and slide a spare cup in before the machine started to dispense coffee. At this stage, I assume he did not know that Cilla was in on the gag – especially since it was Cilla that he was buying the coffee for.

Deviously, Cilla and I agreed on one further ruse: we decided we would tape up the Perspex door with Sellotape... and with great expectation, awaited the outcome.

Finally, he arrived in reception and approached the machine to get Cilla a coffee. Money in... no cup appears... so as quick as a flash, before trying the Perspex door, he produced a spare cup – he then tried the door, which to his amazement didn't move, and a whole cup of coffee is wasted.

He went mad, kicking the machine and swearing at it! From my hiding place, I could see Cilla at the switchboard unable to control her laughter!

She told me later that she had actually wet herself laughing!

Unable to speak, the switchboard remained unanswered, and it resembled a Christmas tree by the time she felt composed enough to answer the calls.'

Once the family moved, Cilla continued her car ferrying for quite a few years to come, but realised that subsidising her wages was mainly due to the poor wage she was receiving at ISR. As a result, in late 1977 she started looking for another better paying job.

Coincidently, her position at ISR was already under review due to changes in technology.

The only problem was that apart from Beaulieu and the Petrochemical Industry, all located in the near vicinity, there was little to nothing else suitable. So she started looking further afield, and Southampton was the most logical area to start her search.

Due to the proposed changes, her boss from ISR, Mr D Woods, gave her the following reference in response to an application she had already made:

'I have been asked by Miss Upson to write to you in respect of her application for employment to your company.

Miss Upson has been employed by ISR as a telephonist/receptionist at Hythe Works for nearly six years. She is now leaving the company following our policy decision to instal (sic) an automatic satellite exchange which makes her position redundant.

During her time with us she has competently handled a PABX3, including seven private wires. This includes the receiving and transmittal of international calls. Her duties also include operation of the Tannoy system for contacting personnel on site and operation of the Telex/Teleprinter apparatus.

Her reception duties involve receiving visitors to the site and their introduction to management, etc.

She is neat in appearance, has a pleasant and sociable manner, and would be well qualified for the position you have in mind.'

On the 11th of October 1977, and armed with several other references – in fact ten years' worth – she had an interview with Roger Young, the personnel officer of a shipping company based in Polygon House, Commercial Road.

On Tuesday the 1st of November 1977, Cilla joined ACLS (Atlantic Container Line Services) as the telephonist/receptionist for the Financial Department. Her annual starting salary was the grand sum of £2,472, plus thirty pence in luncheon vouchers per each working day. Importantly, another benefit of working at ACLS was her enrolment into BUPA, which would be extensively used by her later in life.

ACLS also had additional offices in Overline House, just over the road and next to Southampton's rail terminus. As the business was expanding, they realised they would soon need to move to more appropriately sized offices. Suitable offices were eventually found in Herbert Walker Avenue in Southampton Docks – ironically through dock gate eight and adjacent to the Post House Hotel, where Godfrey Davis was once located. The new buildings had previously been vacated by Union Castle Line, and consisted of two blocks divided into three departmental units.

Paradoxically, and unknown to us both at the time, Cilla and I shared quite a few links during our past lives. In this case, my father worked for Union Castle Line, and frequently called into these offices over the years. Also, Jack the maintenance man at ACLS, actually knew my father from years gone by.

Anyhow, once again, Cilla found herself central and the hub of attention, and astonishingly, an eventual and unexpected house move was just about to make things much easier for her.

Being an international company, ACLS received many foreign visitors, some fleetingly, and other staying for many months, even years.

Amongst them, was Thomas Bengtsson – who cannot be ignored in Cilla's life story as he played a big part in our hectic social life. Thomas was, as you can guess from his name, Scandinavian; Swedish to be exact. At six foot six inches tall, he was always visible, and from his booming laughter, he certainly could not be ignored. He was a natural born joker and would often sport a badge which stated: *'Don't Ask, I'm 6' 6'''*

Although Thomas and I were only one year minus one day apart in age, it appeared that he adopted Cilla and me as surrogate parents. Along with his fellow compatriot, Kjell, he would often spend evenings with us that typically extended well into the early hours of the mornings.

As a practical joker, Thomas once left our house and, for some unknown reason, decided to take our front gate home for the night... If there was a party, then between Cilla and Thomas they would keep everything interesting throughout and beyond. One memorable occasion saw Thomas convincingly dress as a Viking, Cilla as a policewoman, and me as a bumble bee... Yes, quite an eclectic combination!

This occasion was organised by the ACLS social committee and included a riverboat shuffle, which consisted of a quick boat trip to the Isle of Wight and back. What made this so memorable was that when we landed on the shores of the Isle of Wight, we all stormed the nearest pub. Thomas led the charge from ship to pub and was, as per usual, first through the door. In true spirit to his jovial nature, he went in holding a plastic sword above his head and shouting, *'The Vikings have landed!'* It was a surprise to me that we were not thrown out as soon as we entered. To add to this, while Thomas was waiting at the bar to be served, a stranger turned to his friend, and according to Thomas said in Swedish, *'Who do these people think they are dressing up as Vikings?'* Thomas, being the sport he was, called the barman over and ordered drinks for the strangers, before turning to them and saying in his native Swedish: *'We conquer all!'*, and laughed raucously.

There was not one person I knew who could not help but like Thomas.

Sadly, Thomas too has left us far too soon. Some eight weeks after Cilla passed, Thomas suffered a massive heart attack and died at his home in Sweden. Despite this tragedy, there is no better comforting thought that between Cilla, John Williams (who you will read about soon), and Thomas Bengtsson, there is one hell of a party going on in 'Asgard's Valhalla'.

Before I move on, I feel that there are far too many coincidences in Cilla's life not to mention this one... almost six months after Cilla passed, I decided I would visit Little Timbers – as it was once know – and met the current owners, Mr & Mrs Copsey. Shortly after the visit I received an e mail from Mr Copsey, which read:

'Hello Steve, as a matter of interest, I worked as a consultant for Atlantic Container Line in the 80's and a lady, I think was the receptionist, mentioned that she lived at Little Timbers. I just wondered if that she perhaps was your wife, as I remember talk of the motor museum. We were chatting while I was waiting to see my ACL friend... but a long time ago now, probably quite wrong. Regards.'

Of course, Mr Copsey was not wrong since this sparked a deep set memory within me and recalled Cilla once casually mentioning that she had recently met the owner of Little Timbers. To further confirm this, I took a photograph of Cilla sitting at her ACLS reception desk to show Mr Copsey. Without prompting and with true conviction, Mr Copsey confirmed Cilla's identity.

Beauty

True to Cilla's wishes, she finally managed to buy her own horse. On the 30th of August 1973, Cilla willingly and knowingly bought a chestnut horse... complete with a hernia. As crazy as that may seem to some, it actually made sense and achieved two things: firstly, she saved the life of a horse that may well have been put down due to the associated time, costs and vet's bills. Secondly, the purchase price was tiny by comparison to other horses of his age. Also, the owner was glad to pass on the costs, since they would not only save money but would get some back. For both parties involved, this appeared to be a win-win situation, and at fourteen hands high, this proved to be the perfect starter horse for Cilla to own.

Already named Bambi, Cilla knew she had to change the name, so within days he became known as Beauty.

Personally, I never understood why Cilla chose Beauty as a name for a male horse and always assumed, in this instance, that her heart led her... although I must admit, in my humble opinion, it did sound better than Bambi.

Immediately, Cilla concentrated on finding accommodation for her Beauty, and through her extensive network of connections and friends, she soon found space. Within days, she rented the use of a shared five-acre field in Dibden Manor for a mere seventy-five pence a week.

The other horse in the field was a mare called Nizzet, which Cilla knew little about. Beauty first appeared nervous in his new surroundings, but it did not take long for the two horses to gel.

So far so good, but now the expenses were going to start in earnest, and this will also explain the full reason why Cilla sought a part-time job.

Over the years, Cilla's father became pivotal in her keeping and maintaining Beauty. On many occasions, he would go to the field and physically help maintain Beauty's upkeep by doing whatever he could. He even managed to obtain cheap straw for twenty pence a bale from somewhere in Mansbridge, near our current house. The straw itself was essential for what was to come, since on professional advice, Cilla knew she would need to stable Beauty for his pending operation.

Once again, her network of friends helped her find a stable within walking distance of the field. Douglas, other family members, and Cilla's boyfriend David all helped clean, sterilise and bed down the stable so the vet, Mr Gould I believe, could operate on Beauty's hernia. Some of the bales of straw were used to act as the buffers necessary to stop Beauty from moving out of position before, during, and after the operation.

Soon the operation was over – within the week of preparations, actually – and after all costs were taken into account, Cilla realised that she was still in-pocket since the overall costs were still much lower than buying a healthy horse on the open market.

Eventually, Beauty was well enough to be ridden, and a certain family member, being the lightest, was the first to ride him. In the interest of Beauty's health, Cilla thought it best to maintain this regime for a while, especially since she was uncertain how much riding Beauty had previously been used to.

It was not long before Cilla decided it was her time to try out Beauty, so she made the necessary preparations. This first effort was not going to go well, and for Cilla it would cause her weeks of pain and discomfort. During the preparations for a gentle trot around the field, Cilla noticed a few wasps flying in the near vicinity and occasionally shooed them off the best she could. Gently Cilla mounted Beauty, and all went well for the first few moments... until suddenly Beauty shrieked and bucked violently. Without previous indications that this was going to happen, Cilla did not prepare herself for an inevitable tumble. Abruptly she was launched head first over the five-bar gate and into the adjacent road, hitting her head as she did so. At first Cilla picked herself up and started to dust herself down, but it soon became apparent that all was not well: within moments she could see everything in double vision and soon started to be sick by the roadside. Fortunately, a passer-by saw what had happened and stopped to help. On advice from the concerned onlooker, Cilla made everything safe and cautiously made her own way home.

The following day she went to work as usual, but it did not take long for her work colleagues to notice that she was having a medical issue. Worried about her condition, she was immediately sent to hospital in a taxi, where it was confirmed that she had concussion. Neck pain and the occasional headache persisted for just over a week, which meant Douglas stepped in and looked after Beauty's daily regime.

Douglas later found a dead wasp squashed into the tack used on the day of Cilla's unfortunate accident, thus confirming the reasons behind the incident.

Following this setback and Beauty's full recovery from the hernia operation, came a few more changes. Eventually more horses joined the field, which did not always make for a happy balance. Unfortunately, not all of the horse owners had their mount's interests at heart and would often leave them unattended for days on end. This left Cilla with both added costs and even lengthier visits to the field. On many occasions, Cilla found herself feeding all the horses and bringing in fresh water more frequently. This certainly was not an ideal situation, and one that she tried to tackle on many occasions. It seems that the longer the other horses stayed, the less time the respective owners were committing to their horses.

There was also another problem with one of the horses. Misty became violent towards the others, especially Beauty. Misty would often bite and kick out at the other horses for no apparent reason. Cilla constantly battled to get things sorted out and ultimately had to resort to contacting the RSPCA due to both the condition of the other horses and their aggressive behaviour. Eventually this issue was resolved and calm once more descended on the field, which meant that Cilla could finally concentrate on riding Beauty.

From the time Cilla purchased Beauty, and until the family eventually moved away from the area, Cilla would not see her bed until at least midnight on a daily basis – although by now this was just as much to do with her extensive relationships at the time.

Incidentally, Cilla's efforts were often supported by some of her closest friends, namely Nigel Pope, whom I have already mentioned, and John Williams. John in particular enjoyed spending time with both horse and his long-established friend Cilla. Between the two of them, they had a companionable understanding and always looked out for each other, both at work and in leisure. This friendship lasted right up to and until John's sad and untimely death due to cancer in the latter days of February 2015.

In reality, they unsuspectingly said their final goodbyes just before Christmas in 2014, when John visited the house for the last time. Even then, and without the knowledge of what was about to happen, their 'farewell' was quite indicative... almost poignant.

On an associated matter where Beauty was concerned, Douglas, as I have already implied, made his final house move. On the 6th of December 1975, and with all suffering from dreadful colds, they eventually moved to 25 Malmesbury Road in Shirley, another suburb in Southampton. The house, a three bedroomed semi-detached, was ideally suited for Douglas and Joyce, especially since Cilla was still living with her parents. Here, Cilla would commute to ISR for the next few years and Douglas would see out his last few working years.

The only other drawback as far as Cilla was concerned, was now the distance between her new home and her beloved Beauty. As far as Beauty was concerned, this move was fine, whilst Cilla was still working at ISR but there were also weekends and holidays to consider.

Nonetheless, it was this house move which made Cilla do the unthinkable: she eventually sold Beauty. Thinking with her brain and not her heart, she logically realised that the imbalance was too great. Being so close to Southampton city centre meant there were few to no options left open to her. Sadly, there were no fields or grazing rights within miles of the new house, and certainly none that she could get too easily. There were also the ever-increasing costs to consider.

So with a heavy heart on the 15th of April 1976, and at a price of £180, she parted company with one of the last links to her most recent past. Of course, Cilla made sure that the purchaser was right for Beauty, although no more contact was made thereafter.

Relationships

A lthough I have already mentioned at least two former relationships, there is no intention by me to reveal anything salacious, so most of this will be a brief outline based on the most important issues sustained in this area of Cilla's life.

Part of Cilla's appeal was her flirtatious manner, and due to this she had no problem with getting men friends. Indeed, when I first met Cilla and before we became involved, she had no less than four boyfriends to hand! Not all of these encounters were sexual, just deep bonded friendships that she kept throughout her life.

Strangely enough, most women never felt threatened by Cilla, which meant that she had an equal amount of female friends, and all of these were people she could rely on in any given situation.

From the tender age of fifteen, Cilla began to seriously explore boyfriends, and like most of the youth at that age, her relationships were both casual and transitory.

Her first serious encounter was with Colin, which would explain something you may have noticed earlier. Between leaving school and starting work at Gardner & Young Ltd, there was a slight, almost indiscernible gap in Cilla's career. To fill that gap I need to explain more.

On the 4th of March 1967, Cilla and her then boyfriend Colin, approached her parents and announced that they wanted to get married in September. This must have been quite a noteworthy day for her parents, especially her father, because as I have already indicated, Cilla was Daddy's little girl, and I can only imagine how he took the news.

However, within eight weeks, and on the 29th of April, Cilla broke off the engagement... but the story did not end there. On the 10th of May, it was confirmed by the family doctor that Cilla was pregnant. Undoubtedly this was something that could not be ignored, and she clearly remembered the two separate conversations she had with her parents when she eventually revealed her news.

She first approached her mother, saying, '*Mum, I'm pregnant!*'

Her mother was remarkably laid back about it... although she did say that Cilla must tell her father herself, as she would not get involved even though she would support her.

With the first hurdle out of the way, she now knew she had to tell her father; she also knew that this would be much more difficult! Taking all the courage she could muster, she approached him and said, '*Dad, I'll come straight to the point... I'm pregnant.*' True enough, her father was not as understanding, and pondered for a while before a slightly heated conversation took place between them. If Cilla remembered anything about this discussion, she kept it to herself, with one exception: her father looked her square in the eye and finished the conversation with this sentence: '*Good god, girl! Why do you think I gave you rabbits?*'

He then turned away and walked to his inner sanctum: the outside shed.

After a period of frostiness, acceptance crept in and, before long, her father was just as busy smocking and knitting baby clothes, as was her mother.

Christmas was fast approaching, and the once slender Cilla now looked, and felt, like an exaggerated balloon. Despite this, it was life as usual until the 20th of December when Joseph Paul Upson was born.

Only now can I reveal that the previously mentioned 'certain family member' who was of a lighter proportion when I was talking about Beauty: was none other than Joseph, and almost immediately after his birth, Douglas and Joyce took control of their new grandson, which allowed an already slender Cilla to return to work.

Following this event, Cilla decided that having a child would not stop her from getting on with life. Indeed, if anything, it propelled her into a slightly hedonistic part of her life.

Cilla had little to do with Colin from that point on, with the exception of a hearing at the Magistrates Court in Hythe regarding the matter of affiliation and associated payments. On the 21st of February 1968, the courts decided that an amount of £2 per week should be awarded for the upkeep of Joe, as he was now known. The award was to be paid weekly until Joe reached the age of eighteen. By then the courts agreed that an amount of £18 had been accrued, and should be paid at £3 a week until the back payments were met.

Surprisingly this case was brought before the courts by Cilla's father, and not by her.

This did nothing to improve their already stretched relationship, and Colin soon decided that he would be better off somewhere else. Within months, he had emigrated to Canada.

I must admit that although I never met Colin face to face, I did speak to him on many occasions by telephone. He always came across as a lovable rogue who lived his life as simply as he could, with as little outside interference as possible. The few photographs he sent Cilla, which always made me smile, confirmed his lifestyle. With a tied back neckerchief covering his head, and a greying ponytail protruding, he looked every part a hippy.

Sadly, Colin died of cancer on 1st of April 2012, a few months before his intended trip back to the UK, where he finally hoped to meet Joe as an adult. Poignantly, a medical check necessary for him to obtain travel insurance for the trip became the catalyst of the diagnosis.

David I have already mentioned, so from here I will move on...

Cilla became very active with many boyfriends, but none more so than Pete. They met at work in January 1975, but there was a catch: he was married. Although this was not the first affair Cilla had had with a married man, it was certainly one to have an impact on her.

His bad boy image had a certain appeal, and he used this to his advantage where women were concerned. He promised Cilla the earth and, by all accounts due to his reputation, he could give it. Here was a man feared by other men and adored by women, since his reputation for violence had been very well documented. Indeed, he had once been described by one poetic observer as: '*A rough diamond hewn from the soul of the Earth.*'

For once, Cilla thought there was a real chance of marriage, save the obvious problem of him already being married. However, February 1976 saw the first of many break-ups, and by April of that year the relationship finally failed. Through stress, this episode caused her to smoke more, and it was only now, unbelievably, after twelve years of being a regular smoker, that her father found out that she smoked. There were no issues relating to this revelation, but it was surprising that Cilla was able to keep this hidden from him for so long.

In these instances, Cilla bounced right back but, unfortunately, she was due a medical wakeup call. Apart from peritonitis, which in itself is extremely unpleasant and dangerous, her next affliction caught everybody by surprise. Once again, I shall bring this up later and in accordance with other illnesses that Cilla was unfortunate enough to suffer.

Anyhow, relationships came and went, but most of these were casual since Cilla now felt that any serious relationship would be too much for her to cope with. Due to this, she unconsciously convinced herself that being unattached was not as bad as she thought it would be, and this gave her the freedom she needed to get on with life.

Now, despite everything I had just said, this is where I come into the picture!

In late October 1979, I met Cilla whilst visiting her offices in the Western Docks, Southampton. By this time, as you now know, Cilla was the switchboard operator for the shipping company, Atlantic Container Line Services. I was visiting the offices at Cilla's request and in my capacity as general manager of *Dock News*, a retail business located just inside dock gate five and within metres of *Titanic*'s departure dock.

I was not looking for a relationship at the time since I was already married and we were expecting my first, and only, child. So, for the story to continue, I must be as open as possible about our meeting and as honest as I can be about the ensuing consequences.

Many staff members from within Cilla's company wanted to have the *Southern Evening Echo* delivered. This practice was not unusual, as my firm supplied every newspaper that was sold within the dock's boundaries, but since we as a company found it almost impossible to employ somebody to do the deliveries, it was left to me to physically involve myself in the task. I enjoyed the freedom of driving from business to business, which also gave me the opportunity to meet up with the many staff involved in the purchase of what was a lucrative venture. In addition, I was always available to top up any dwindling stocks of *Early Evening Echo's* at our various shops, especially when there was a current hot story to be read.

Ironically, I met my then boss, Alan Blondel, through my first wife Lin, who frequently babysat for his son.

Immediately Cilla and I struck up a strong rapport and found that our interests were similar. We certainly had a lot in common. From that first meeting I looked forward to visiting her offices, and my time spent there extended beyond the level it should have. We talked of many things, and during those chats I started to get the feeling that Cilla was interested in me. However, she came across as being sophisticated and in truth, I always saw Cilla as a class above me and could never have imagined anything more than mere chatter.

Over time, our newfound affiliation appeared static, but with unexpected outside influences that was about to change. What appeared to be the catalyst to our relationship transformation was, surprisingly, a discussion Cilla had with one of the four male friends I alluded to earlier. Apparently, as she told me a few years later, my name came up frequently when she was with this one particular friend. Even if Cilla did not immediately notice, her close friends soon realised that she had subconsciously revealed certain affections for me. Indeed, her boyfriend even felt it necessary to mention the point, and went one stage further by suggesting that she should do something about it and *'get him out of your system.'* With this prompt, her immediate reaction was to take his advice.

Unbeknownst to me, she carefully planned her next move, and this she did by inviting me to her house to help her with a small structural problem with an internal wall. My interest towards her was not as immediate as she had expected, and further structural problems needed seeing to... What happened next came straight out of the opening scene from David Lean's classic film, *'Brief Encounter'*.

On reflection, I am not quite sure what I was thinking since, as I have already said, I had a child on the way and I always considered Cilla exclusively above me, but as our relationship gradually developed and the visits increased... I am not ashamed to say that I eventually succumbed to her charms.

Her passion for life and passion for love surpassed everything I had previously experienced. My intensity in the relationship soon exceeded that of Cilla's, and I became besotted without thought of the consequences. On Cilla's part, it was if she had found what she was finally looking for, and told me soon afterwards that there would be no one else in her life. True to her word, she immediately stopped seeing her regular men friends and became devoted to our newfound relationship.

By now, I had a beautiful son named Adrian, but I had to make a life changing choice... and I had to ask myself one question: What now was the right thing to do? Of course, I could do the most honourable thing and stay with my wife and son... or consider the alternative.

I have the deepest respect for my ex-wife Lin, and I cannot blame her for anything that followed – indeed, when seeking a divorce my solicitor chastened me for not helping him enough with the proceedings, and in that instance was unable to provide him with any wrongdoings on her part. My logic, if you could call it that, for the departure from our marriage was simplistic and, perhaps, a bit too analytical for the situation. The way I saw it, by leaving a wife and new-born son so soon after birth meant that when my son grew up he would know no different. As it later turned out, this hard-hearted rationale proved right, as Lin eventually remarried and my son and I bonded exponentially... to confirm this point and happily, we still have a wonderful relationship to this day. This situation has recently help me through many a dark moment!

Personally, I feel this next point really needs to be said, and I can think of no better way of putting it. Truly, Lin's husband Andy is one of the nicest, caring and most thoughtful men I have ever had the pleasure to meet. Likewise, Lin has my utter respect, especially for the way she acted under the circumstances both then and now. Happily, Lin even met Cilla on several occasions and showed no animosity towards her or the enforced situation she once found herself in. Eventually, Lin and Andy went on to have a son of their own, and even now, the closeness of Adrian and his brother Daniel is astoundingly fraternal and solid.

Following my divorce, Cilla and I married on the 16th of September 1982. Fatefully – and of course we were unaware of this fact at the time – due to PSP, Cilla was within weeks of the halfway point in her life... It is only now that I ponder this thought.

Now we enter a new chapter in Cilla's life, and one that was as familiar to her as it would have been to her parents.

Unbeknownst to me, and thanks to some form of intervention from my newfound mother-in-law, following a short interview on the 9th of May 1983, I landed a job at Beaulieu as Administrator to The National Motor Museum Trust. This was a newly created post to assist the curator, Michael Ware, regarding all administrative issues.

Fortunately for me, and as this was a new position, within reason, I was able to mould it around my own abilities. This position also gave Michael Ware the freedom he needed to concentrate on more important issues.

Indeed, I vividly remember Michael once introducing me to a guest as the person *'who allows me to play with old cars.'* If truth be told, this was the best job I had ever had, and the location was second to none. The pay was low but somehow expected since I was now working for a charity, and furthermore, who could resist the setting right in the heart of the New Forest? I also remember the last paragraph of my job description: *'Direct liaison with Lord Montagu relating to overseas rallies, sponsorship and other Trust related work.'* It was this paragraph that always made me think how proud my late father-in-law would have been.

Even now, I remember how privileged I was to be following him in his footsteps... I still recall how lucky and proud I felt on my first day there.

To make things more interesting, Michael Ware spent his whole working life in and around the veteran, vintage and the classic car world, and from 1963 he joined Beaulieu as photographer and photographic librarian. This meant that he knew and had at some point worked closely alongside Douglas.

During my tenure, I was fortunate enough to mix with royalty and, like Cilla, stars of stage and screen. Astonishingly, and to Cilla's satisfaction, I even appeared in several of the Beaulieu television adverts, as well as on various posters and in pamphlets!

In my capacity as administrator, I also got heavily involved with 'special' guests, and often accompanied them to different locations or assisted them in other ways: Prince Philip, Lord Snowden, Denis Thatcher, Prince and Princess Michael of Kent, Murray Walker, Patrick Macnee, Fiona Fullerton, Fred Dinenage, Val Doonican, Bamber Gascoigne, Fern Britton, Judith Chalmers, Jody Scheckter, Martin Brundle, Peter Ustinov and Richard Noble to name a few. At the numerous shows I attended, I also escorted people like David Essex, Ralph Bates, Peter Blake, Bob Monkhouse, Cliff Richard and many, many others who found themselves around our various stands at motor shows.

Inevitably, Cilla would be with me on more formal occasions, and two in particular come to mind.

An evening event held at the Sheraton Park Hotel on Thursday the 11th of October 1984 had been organised by Kerry de Courcy, the Champagne entrepreneur in Lord Montagu's honour. I was there in my official capacity, along with Cilla, as a guest of Kerry.

At one point, I left Cilla to her own devices and mingled accordingly. Later in the evening I sought her out, and soon found her in deep conversation with the actor Hugh Lloyd and his lovely wife Shan. Both Cilla and Hugh were smoking, and along with Shan, were having a whale of a time – such was Cilla's charm.

Her charms were to be extended further that evening, as towards the end of the function, Cilla and I were unexpectedly invited to an after party dinner. The dinner turned out to be much more formal than I had anticipated, since the table was predominately occupied by Lords of the realm. Apart from Lord Montagu, there was also Lord 'Peter' Nelson, Lord Bernard Delfont and several others. The reason I have singled out Lord 'Peter' Nelson and Lord Bernard Delfont is because Cilla was sitting between them. Significantly, I was sitting opposite Cilla, and next to Lord David Strathcarron – best known as the "motorcycling peer" – but still well within earshot of her conversations. Here, Cilla used all her natural charm, skill and extensive wit to have both of her immediate companions enthralled. In true fashion, she did not hold back from asking the many questions we all would have liked to have asked given the same opportunity. There was lots of laughter coming from this quarter, and looking around, I swear that some of the remaining guests wished they were more involved. From where I was sitting, from either side of Cilla I could hear names being bandied about like Frank Sinatra, Shirley Bassey, Judy Garland, Eartha Kitt, Benny Hill, Tony Hancock and, of all people, Lady Emma Hamilton.

Apart from the laughter, the remaining conversations were often muted, and I shall now explain why.

Now here is the irony of this particular anecdote, and one I have deliberately held back to the end of this specific story. Sitting well within earshot of Cilla's conversations was another well-known guest, and someone who now serves an eternal association with her; here, Nigel Dempster made a point of being unobtrusive, and almost appeared invisible to some of the other guests. He made no fuss about his attendance, and almost blended into the background. However, he was more than intrigued with what was being said around him, and appeared to be taking countless mental notes. At one point, I had to interrupt a certain exchange of information between Cilla and her charmed audience to formerly introduce him to her. Once introduced, Cilla turned the tables on him and began to ask him many a question. Nigel certainly seemed intrigued by her persistence, and told her that she should come and work with him.

What made this meeting of minds so extraordinary, was that Nigel too would eventually develop and die of complications due to PSP. But believe it or not, his connection to PSP had all but escaped me until quite recently when I came across an article highlighting his sad death and the cause.

To clarify Nigel's credentials, at the time he was a revered *Daily Mail* columnist and, like Cilla, a prolific diarist. He was once described as '*the hot-breathed newspaper gossip ace of his day.*' Despite Cilla's persistence, I am almost certain there was nothing newsworthy from that night for him to add to his upcoming column... and I am sure he had heard it all before.

Nigel, as I have already said, eventually lost his life to associated complications arising from PSP on 12th of July 2007.

Much like Dudley Moore, here is a link to an interview about Nigel's life with PSP and, once more, I urge you to view this to the very end.

https://www.youtube.com/watch?v=4hhE_qvA5tQ

I clearly remember the trip home from London that night, and on the way I asked Cilla if she had any gossip for me. Her simple response was both telling and characteristic of her as a person: *'That is between me and the bedpost.'* She then gave her typical raucous laugh, before falling asleep.

The other event where she completely enthralled her table companion was held at the Post House Hotel, (formerly the Skyway Hotel and later the Holiday Inn), where Cilla already had a strong association.

One month prior to the Sheraton Park Hotel event, on Saturday the 15th of September 1984, we were formally invited to a special lunch at the Southampton Boat Show – Ironically, the Internationally renowned Southampton Boat Show, is now known as the PSP Southampton Boat Show after the sponsors, Premier Shipping and Packing Limited.

At first I could not find our table, but I looked up and saw Cilla waving to me from her seated position. Once again I sat opposite her, although this time we were on a round table and I was less involved with her conversations.

I would have liked to have been closer since she was sitting next to Sir Alec Rose.

All I remember was that they lagged behind the rest of us during the meal, and we all had to wait patiently because they always appeared to be deep in conversation. The waitress at one point started clearing the table from my side while she waited for Cilla and Sir Alec to finish!

There were more events and more stars over the years, but all this came to an end when I changed career in December 1988. I was truly sad to leave Beaulieu and will be forever thankful for the opportunity they and my mother-in-law had given me. My career change meant that glamour was going to be a thing of the past, but I still had Cilla – and that was the most defining feature.

Sadly, Cilla's mother Joyce developed breast cancer and eventually vacated her flat in Gosport before moving in with us. This was the first time we as a couple had had to deal with hands-on caring. Due to work commitments, I had less to do with the situation, but by now Cilla had left work due to voluntary redundancy and ill health. Sadly, on the 16th of June 1993, Joyce passed away aged eighty-four in Southampton's General Hospital, where Cilla finally passed. We eventually made two house moves following this, before finally settling in West End on the outskirts of Southampton.

As far as relationships go, Cilla's experiences were undeniably defined by diversity, and this was something that enriched her very being. Yet, despite several setbacks and heartaches over the years, she never regretted a moment of her life in love or anything else that life threw at her.

Typically Cilla

I hope so far that you have realised we have been talking about one incredible person here. Her zest for existence, and her ability to live life to the full was apparent, and appeared to be genetically encoded into her life's blood.

I also hope you fully appreciate her selflessness. I can simply sum this up, by quoting the contents of a letter I found, circa 1956:

'Nov 21st

Little Timbers
Fair Oak

Dear Father Xmas please will you by (sic) *me a cowgirl outfit. And a brides outfit for my best walkie-talkie doll. And a pair of wellingtons for her.*

I am seven years old. and (sic) *I hope you have a happy christmas* (sic)*. xx oo xx oo xx oo. with* (sic) *all my love from Priscilla'*

The most defining picture I drew from this short note was her forward-thinking, notably evident by the date, and truly unselfish attitude, since the items requested were not directly for her.

In essence, Cilla grew up into someone we would all like to be: spontaneous, genuine, sincere, relaxed, funny and open, and astonishingly, this all came to her naturally.

She was extremely generous in many ways, and had a natural aptitude of putting people at ease in any given situation. Humour was another instinctive and significant feature, which she used to good effect to disarm the most hostile of those we often meet in life. Her infectious laughter was even heard throughout the very corridors of power, and beyond; at one time, even the Usher during a private visit to the House of Lords noted it.

She never feared living life to the full, and always hauled others less willing along with her. Certainly, Cilla never went to dull parties because parties only really started when she arrived! People often referred to hearing Cilla's distinctive laughter and knew that, once heard, all would be well.

Her strength of character was once defined by her standing up against a known bully, and ripping to shreds his barrister when the situation eventually ended up in court. During the incident concerned, she had single-handedly put herself between the bully, his dog – which had badly bitten her friend's arm at his behest – and her wounded and frightened companion. Alone, she literally stood her ground both then and later in court. She even had the court tittering at her 'off the cuff' remarks, which were often barbed and expressive. From then on, there was little doubt about the final outcome of the case... He was found guilty as charged, thanks to Cilla's unwavering and conclusive evidence.

Likewise, her effortless generosity, especially toward animals, was not only defined by her actions but was also well documented. It was generally known that there were animals that lived well beyond their own natural life because of her accomplishments. I remember her spending hours, nights, and days, on hard floors to help and encourage one of our beloved pets through a crisis. The only reason they pulled through was due to her devotion and expertise in understanding what was required beyond medicine. In our life together, and roughly calculated over the years, there were eight dogs, two hamsters, one canary and twelve cats that owned Cilla's affections. Of course, the list does not even include one horse and the various animals Cilla had as a child on the family smallholding in Fair Oak. Moreover, during this time, not once did she let them down, or did she divert her attentions away from them when they most needed it.

She also inherited her father's green fingers and loved gardening, which is still apparent by the many plants, trees and shrubs still living in our garden now. It was her belief that gardening was a privilege given to the world, and that every plant and flower ever grown in a garden was only a weed accepted by society. This meant she often cultivated some plants not normally recognised by others as being acceptable. She had no particular favourites, but I do know that one of the last words she ever spoke was Hyacinths.

True to character, she would seek out the weak and give them an equal chance in life, even at her own expense. As later in life, and even in the direst of situations, she would ask after others above herself. Indeed, it was another one of her most significant features!

Well Travelled

There is one area I have only just touched on, but it is important enough to share with you right now. In her lifetime, Cilla was relatively well travelled, and from this she expanded her knowledge which, in turn, helped me in my understanding of the wider world.

Despite me spending three years working on a private yacht in the Mediterranean as a deck boy, and visiting at least fifteen counties myself, culturally I never felt as well travelled.

Cilla changed all that.

For instance, I have now driven on foreign soil more times than I can remember. However, the first time I ever drove abroad Cilla was by my side, encouraging me and helping me build my confidence. She also helped me embrace different cultures, especially where food was concerned. In Sweden, for example, she already knew many of the correct and accepted practices despite it also being her first visit. She knew this because she had read and studied everything she needed to know to survive beyond our shores.

Her various travels took her to America, Canada, Bermuda, Bahamas, Cayman Islands, Sweden, Denmark, France, Germany, Belgium, Holland, Monte Carlo, Switzerland, Italy, Spain and Greece. But none held her heart quite like somewhere a little nearer to home: Guernsey!

Guernsey was like a second home to Cilla, and was where her mother Joyce was born. Joyce was, along with hundreds of other children, forced to flee Guernsey in fear of invasion during the First World War, and travelled by boat to Portsmouth. She was just eight years old. Here, the family eventually split into several groups and were sent to different parts of the United Kingdom. Joyce, for some reason, initially stayed in the Portsmouth area... and the rest, as they say, is history.

Our eventual trips to Guernsey were many, which included our *first* honeymoon! This 'happy mistake' was due to an oversight on my part, as I had booked the honeymoon to commence directly after our wedding, which seems logical. Unfortunately, I had misunderstood essential paperwork as well as miscalculating the dates. The honeymoon itself eventually arrived two weeks ahead of the actual wedding due to this administrative error. So we ended up having two honeymoons... but who was complaining? I certainly wasn't!

Anyhow, back to Guernsey... excitedly, and like a school kid, she dragged me around the various sights – and some places tourists do not normally venture. She took me to her late uncle's house, Le Preaux, La Route De Sausmarez in St. Martin's. Not satisfied with merely pointing out the tree where her uncle had hidden the family's treasure when they were eventually invaded during World War Two, she actually persuaded me to knock on the door and asked the resident if we could look around. Surprisingly, the owners were more than happy to do this after Cilla eventually told her of the connection.

Incidentally, whilst reading details of properties on the Island, I noticed the house had recently sold for £3.8 million.

Fortunately, and during the earliest stages of her illness, she and her cousin Lindy took a trip down memory lane by taking a well-earned break back to Guernsey, which they both enjoyed immensely.

I would now like to take a backward step here and mention my most recent findings, which I am sure you will most certainly find interesting.

During her various travels she sent many a postcard home, and I have recently unearthed two which I found particularly amusing. What first amazed and delighted me about the cards was how much information she managed to squeeze onto them! These relate to a European trip Cilla and her friend Ellen took in 1969. I have included them here to further show her resilience and sense of adventure.

In date order:

'Dear Mum, Dad and Jo (sic)*, As you can see, we are in Switzerland and it is 7.0 am* (sic) *Sunday morning. So far it hasn't stopped raining, but we haven't got wet because we have been in various cars. We have had a television interviewer, a movie director, a flying instructor and a famous racing driver. All have been very courteous and have brought* (sic) *us coffees etc. I have only spent 2 francs so far. We slept on a mountain side last night. I was very worried last night when Ellen*

disappeared over the edge thinking it was the path. Over she went rucksack and all. I really wet myself laughing when I found out she was alright. She grazed her hand but is otherwise alright. We are by Lake Geneva at the moment and still giggling about last night. It is very beautiful here, with the mountains etc. In a moment we are setting off for Italy and have just realised that we know no Italian whatsoever. Still!!! We are warm, dry and having a lovely time, so don't worry. We also had a lift in a bread van yesterday and the driver gave us a bag of hot fresh rolls. They were lovely and we had them with chicken & cheese. Everything is so nice and the propritress (sic) (female proprietor) *of this café has just told us she will post the cards for us. Be good. I miss you all. Look after my little Jo* (sic). *See you soon. Lots of LUV* (sic) *Cilla.'*

Although not relevant, this card alone tells its own story, and I was soon left wondering who the 'famous racing driver' was, so I cross-referenced the card to her diary of that year. Her diary does not reveal much more information, but does highlight the fact that the car was a souped-up NSU. As an automotive racing fan, I cannot imagine who in the world that could have been, other than perhaps a specific German driver I have in mind! Cilla gave no indication of his nationality, so I shall continue guessing and keep my thoughts to myself.

Anyhow, the next postcard links nicely, and appeared to immediately follow the first one:

'Dear Mum, Dad and Jo (sic). *As you see we are now in Milan Italy. We were a bit stuck in a small village in the Swiss mountains yesterday but a kind garage owner took us in and out of the rain and gave us a lunch of steak and spaghetti. He then paid for a taxi to take us to the main autoroute for Italy. We couldn't believe his kindness! We then got a car which later picked up two Norwegian girl hitchhikers, we found them in the snow – yes snow! – in the Alps. They were frozen. They had had trouble with a lift and had to jump for it. She brought us straight across the border to Milan where we stayed last night in a youth hotel with the Norwegian girls. It was very clean and very cheap and we feel very refreshed this morning. This city is very beautiful with fountains and statues etc etc. Now it is blazing hot. So far we have seen rain, rain and snow, especially crossing the Alps. We went through the Simplon tunnel. Wow! But the scenery was fantastic and our ears went pop at the high altitude. Still as I say now we have hit the hot*

weather and after our breakfast will head for Monte Carlo. Miss you all. Look after my little Jo (sic). *Love Cilla xxx.'*

Incredibly, it is almost as if I could picture their journey from the brief outline of the two postcards. There was drama, excitement and adventure captured on each of the cards, almost as if their only purpose was to be relayed here in Cilla's life's story.

In life we sometimes focus so much on tomorrow that we forget to live for today; that was certainly not the case where Cilla was concerned, especially where a chance to travel appeared. Ironically, the only thing that could possibly tie her down would be an illness that restricted movement.

Now, please read on to learn more about the person who was full of character and expectation, because we are now entering a realm of certainty and finality.

Cilla's Medical History

D espite everything I have mentioned up and until now, Cilla did have a troubled medical life, and I have already mentioned a medical wakeup call. Before I move on to the complexities of Cilla's illnesses over the years, and finally moving on to PSP, I need to highlight how she dealt with her prior medical issues.

1968

Although I cannot be certain of the correct date or year, possibly 1968, Cilla developed peritonitis. While recuperating at home from an unknown minor illness, she became extremely uncomfortable due to severe pain and vomiting. Being all alone in the house meant she had to haul herself along the landing on her hands and knees before negotiating the stairs to call for help... And after an agonisingly long wait, help finally arrived!

At one stage, her condition was said to be touch or go, since it was apparent she was close to contracting sepsis. Even after the removal of her appendix and the associated discharge, the wound had to be left open for regular treatment. Packed with cotton wool and gauze, the wound was repeatedly flushed out and repacked over a long period of time. Eventually, the wound was sealed and allowed to heal. I do remember her being self-conscious of the deep scar this left.

1974

1974 was the first time Cilla complained of lower back problems. Naturally, and at the time, Cilla was not thinking long-term when this occurred.

1976

Now for the aforementioned medical wakeup call... In the early days of March 1976, Cilla was feeling tired and slightly depressed. She put this down to her hectic lifestyle and resisted going to the doctor until the 15th of March. Following an internal exam, the doctor concluded that there was a potential problem and arranged for Cilla to be seen again. Surprisingly, her next visit was not at the surgery but at the Royal South Hants Hospital. Here, she was shocked to hear that there were cancerous cells found and she would need a dilatation and curettage (D & C). Simply put, under general anaesthetic, she would have selective tissue removed from her womb.

Anxiously she waited for the inevitable day, which was not confirmed until Thursday the 8th of April when a letter arrived. She had a further anxious wait, since the date on the letter confirming the procedure was for the 22nd of April. Cilla was finally given her pre-med at 8.00am on the 23rd, and soon after removed from the ward to the theatre.

By all accounts, the procedure went well and by the 24th, she was discharged into the care of her parents. Although she fully recovered, it was something that consistently played on her mind. She had regular checks thereafter, which would later result in more surgery. A final 'all clear' was given in 1978.

1982

The regular checks I mentioned resulted in the following. In June of 1982, and just prior to our wedding in September, Cilla had a laparoscopic bilateral sterilisation. If we ever considered having children, then due to this procedure and despite the D & C, the decision was irrefutably taken away from us.

It is strange to think that following this procedure, we never actually spoke of having children – although both felt blessed to have had our own through separate relationships.

1983

Following her sterilisation, and with continual problems due to heavy periods and strong period pains, Cilla once more sought medical help.

Initially, she thought back to her days of cancer and expressed her concerns to her doctor.

Without second thought, the doctor arranged a total abdominal hysterectomy NEC.

Of course, there are always consequences to these procedures, and this was going to be no different. Normally, menopause happens because a woman's ovaries stop producing the hormones oestrogen and progesterone. Furthermore, menopause usually occurs around the forty-five to fifty-year age group. In Cilla's case, and at the age of thirty-four, it hit hard... really, really hard. In effect, she eventually ended up with three of the usually diagnosed symptoms associated with menopause and, thankfully no more. These were hot flushes, including night sweats, subtle mood swings, and trouble sleeping. None of these were easy to live with, especially in somebody with Cilla's habitual upbeat nature. After experimenting with various prescribed drugs, the symptoms were mostly kept under control – although sometimes this was difficult due to other problems, which included continual back pain.

Thinking back, Cilla always suffered from trouble with sleeping and mostly took prescribed pills to help in this matter. This issue would also play its part in Cilla's wellbeing, and will be addressed later.

1986

On the 1st of December, Cilla was signed off work for almost a month due to a ruptured spinal cord. There was no known or apparent reason, or blow to her back for this to have happened, other than some casual clearing of the garden area.

At some time during this period, Cilla suffered from, in non-technical language, policeman's heel, or correctly known – plantar fasciitis. Policeman's heel is known to be the most common cause of pain in the heel. People affected by plantar fasciitis will feel pain in the sole of the foot, and in the heel. The pain tends to be particularly severe in the morning, especially when taking the first few steps after waking up. This was the case when Cilla started walking after long periods of rest. The pain and stiffness in the foot is mainly due to weight-bearing and often caused Cilla to limp. From memory, this only affected her right foot – I say from memory, because Cilla spent many years in a wheelchair before she died.

1987

Cilla saw a specialist at BUPA's private hospital in Sarum Road for initial tests on her back, and later had scans. The scans were quite revealing and showed further spinal damage, which they decided to deal with through a series of injections. It would take another year before more drastic surgical measures were finally taken.

As a side issue, Cilla's specialist at the hospital was an expert orchid grower, which interested her greatly, so much so that Cilla also started to cultivate orchids.

1988

Back pain, in my humble opinion, may well have had something to do with her association with Beauty, and in particular with her concussive fall in 1973.

Fortunately, and with the help of our health insurance, we used an opportunity in 1988 to seek necessary medical advice. Firstly, as per protocol, it was necessary for Cilla to attend an appointment with her GP. From here, we waited less than a week before being referred to a specialist.

Following numerous tests, X-rays and scans, Cilla was scheduled for back surgery and on the 6th of January 1988 she had a spinal fusion between L5 and S1.

Sadly, and most understandably, any physical relationship within the marriage was practically over due to this and all the ensuing problems Cilla was to endure. This by no means is meant as a complaint, just a practical observation that I feel is worth mentioning. It is also a reminder that love and sex, in these instances, can be separated by a realistic understanding within any relationship.

1989

In December of 1988, we were extremely fortunate to be invited to one of Cilla's oldest friend Ellen's wedding in Canada – You may well recall the exploits of Cilla and her friend Ellen when they travelled through Europe.

The happy occasion was to take place in May of 1989, so we gratefully accepted. To make this trip worthwhile, we decided that nothing less than a three-week trip was viable. As a result of some financial assistance from Cilla's Mother, coupled with our forward-thinking and planning, we finally arrived in wintery conditions a week before the wedding.

Graciously, Ellen and John invited Cilla to be their chief bridesmaid and official witness in their wonderful ceremony.

Throughout our time there, we saw winter and spring conditions arrive and go in quick succession. The summer weather, in the latter week-and-a-half, consisted of temperatures in the mid to high-eighties. The reason I am mentioning this is because of something Cilla suggested we do together while there... white water rafting! I pointed out that she was in no real fit state to do this, but her determination for fun overrode my fears. This was an adventure I shall never forget, and if at any point it affected Cilla in the negative then she kept it to herself. I have always admired her for her gutsy and adventurous spirit, but in this instance, I never really felt comfortable when thinking of her fragile back.

Anyhow, putting that aside, Cilla later in the year struggled with pain in her knees. What started out as a diagnostic arthroscopy of the knee, ended up with the scraping of the articular cartilage. The subsequent scarring on Cilla's knees had a major impact on her life. Cilla always considered her legs as one of her most defining features – although, in truth, she had the 'whole package' as some of her many admirers would verify. For months and months following the operation, she preferred to keep her knees covered.

It was also confirmed later in this year that Cilla was registered physically disabled due to her ongoing and extensive musculoskeletal issues.

1990

In May, Cilla underwent a laminectomy.

During this procedure, the back muscles are set aside rather than cut, and the parts of the vertebra adjacent to the lamina are usually left intact. Recovery from a laminectomy usually occurs within a few days following surgery, but Cilla took a lot longer, which could have been due to her previous bouts of surgery.

To make matters worse, in June Cilla ended up back in hospital. Here, again, she needed surgery – although this time she had a discectomy. A discectomy is the surgical removal of herniated disc due to material pressing on a nerve root or the spinal cord itself. Unfortunately, this procedure involves removing the central portion of an intervertebral disc.

1990 proved to be a dire year for Cilla, as once more she had to endure surgery. In August, following more invasive tests, she needed another laminectomy. It was now, I believe, that she had metal rods and pins inserted to both strengthen her back and to protect the surgery.

1993

In February, we were invited to Harley Street to see another independent back specialist. Although these trips became regular for a while, what made this trip so different was what happened afterwards. We had just left the specialist's office and pulled away from our parking spot. Understandably, I was slightly distracted as Cilla was quite emotional due to discussions of further procedures. However, I suddenly became aware of movement to my right. I braked hard and barely missed a man in a grey suit who had run from my right and straight into the path of my car. The man half-turned and waved as a form of apology, before sprinting to a taxi he had just waved down. Once again the man turned and made his apologies as he waved yet again. It was only then that we realised it was none other than Gary Lineker. I said to Cilla afterwards that we had been within a fraction-of-an-inch of ending the career of one of Britain's most well-known football stars!

The net result of these trips to Harley Street was that in March, Cilla had more injections into her facet joints in King Edward VII's Hospital in Sussex. This, apparently, was due to a noticeable degeneration.

The following month, Cilla required more work at King Edward VII's Hospital, this time on her sacroiliac. The sacroiliac is a joint between the lower spine (sacrum) and the hipbone (ileum). Here, they performed a procedure known as cryoanalgesia. The cryoneurolysis, as it is also known, is a procedure where liquid nitrogen is directly administered to a specific area. The idea is to freeze the affected tissue or nerve ending in order to stimulate its regeneration.

1994

The theme continued throughout October and November of this year, where Cilla endured yet another set of procedures at King Edward VII's Hospital. Here, she tolerated a series of epidurals. An Epidural is a technique that frequently involves injections of drugs through a catheter placed into the epidural space. The injections were supposed to result in a temporary loss of sensation, which includes the sensation of pain. This occurs by blocking the transmission of signals through nerve fibres in or near the spinal cord. Sadly, these were much less effective than perhaps they should have been.

1995

The month of February was virtually taken up by epidural techniques and steroid injections in various joints. Once more, the location for the procedures was King Edward VII Hospital, which Cilla liked as a venue, but intensely disliked the reasons for going there. Despite her feelings, she very rarely made public her aversion to the various practices that were, by virtue of degenerative discs, and enforced upon her.

1996

Not all of Cilla's more recent woes came from back pain.

In March, Cilla suffered a trip and, as a result, fractured the metatarsal base in which one of the metatarsals became displaced from the tarsus. The metatarsal bones are a group of five long bones in the foot, located between the tarsal bones of the hind, mid-foot and the phalanges of the toes. These series of bones lack individual names, so the metatarsal bones are numbered from the side of the great toe. On charts, the first, second, third, fourth and fifth metatarsal are often depicted with Roman numerals.

The impact did disrupt her then slow-healing back, which meant the enforced rest needed to work for both foot and back.

By the way, most footballers will be aware of this predicament, because it is a common injury sustained in their field of work. This, perhaps, is the first of a few unintentional puns, so please bear with me.

1998

1998 was a quiet year for Cilla, as she only had one visit to Kind Edward VII Hospital. Once again, she had an epidural. However, this was to be her last visit to that particular hospital, since the specialist felt that he could do no more for her. Despite this, her back problems were not quite over.

It was during this time, and while reflecting on her previous illnesses, that she began to think about the future, in particular her up and coming fiftieth year, which is when she suggested I plan something to celebrate. To give the celebrations some form of weight, I shall cover this story later.

1999

In Cilla's case, medically it appeared everything went wrong, and this year proved no different. In March, Cilla was sent to the private Chalybeate Hospital (now the Spire Southampton Hospital), for a liver test, which immediately came back as abnormal.

In May, Cilla was formerly diagnosed with alcoholic hepatitis, which simply put is inflammation of the liver due to excessive intake of alcohol. It is usually found in association with a fatty liver, and an early sign of alcoholic liver disease. Without immediate attention, this problem may contribute to the progression of fibrosis, leading to cirrhosis. Signs and symptoms of alcoholic hepatitis include jaundice, fluid accumulation in the abdominal cavity and fatigue. At this stage, hepatic encephalopathy, or brain dysfunction due to liver failure was a major cause for concern. Mild cases can be self-limiting, and in severe cases, have a high risk of death. In some severe cases, it can be treated with glucocorticoids.

I remember sitting with Cilla and holding her hand as the doctor explained the condition and what was then the necessary course of action. The doctor, from my memory, called it a 'bright liver' but gave Cilla hope when he said that if she stopped drinking, then the liver could repair itself. In fact, he went one stage further and even told Cilla that the alternative was a limited life, which could be as short as three months. Whether this was a shock tactic or not, I am unsure, but it was certainly an effective measure.

Given the alternative, Cilla decided there and then to stop drinking. From that day forth, she never touched another alcoholic drink or was even tempted by others to drink – and unbelievably, some tried hard to persuade her! In these instances, Cilla was never shy about talking to others about this condition, and quickly laughed off their offers. Indeed, it came up in conversation far too frequently, since many people remarked on Cilla drinking non-alcoholic drinks when we went out.

It is true, Cilla used alcohol to excess, but this was not behind her inherent abilities in having fun. By stopping drinking, you would imagine that her outlook on life would have changed, perhaps even that she would have become withdrawn and possibly consider not socialising. No... She was having none of it. Especially since by not drinking the process failed to decrease her powers of having fun or make her shrink away from public view. Truly this proved that the strong character within did not need stimulants to improve her social abilities or to enhance her entertaining skills.

As it turned out, an ensuing test proved her liver had actually reverted back to normal and was fully functioning once more.

While I am on this subject, I must mention a short story relevant to her ability to drink in quantity. Obviously, the following incident took place well before she was diagnosed with a problem with her liver.

As a non-drinker I was given a bottle of vodka from somebody knowing no different. Understanding Cilla's capacity for alcohol, I decided to hide the bottle until I thought a celebration was due and would present it accordingly. That day eventually arose, and when the time was right I announced to all and sundry that I had, in a very safe place, a bottle and I would get it straight away. Cilla looked at me and said, *'No you haven't.'*

I begged to differ, and proceeded to walk next door from our neighbour's house to retrieve the bottle. Before I could take another step, Cilla repeated her statement: *'No you have not!'*

I stopped in my tracks and said, *'I have a bottle of vodka which I have been saving for such an occasion and it is well hidden.'*

Cilla came back with her final reply: *'No... what you have is a bottle of water... I found that bottle months ago.'*

Now, before I move on, I want to raise one very important issue that some of you might think relates Nigel Dempster, Dudley Moore and Cilla together: alcohol!

Nigel Dempster was once quoted as being, *'fond of a drink'*, and had a *'liking for a bottle of wine or three'*, and after once appearing in a state of dishevelment, it was wrongly assumed that he had drunk himself under the table the night before. Either way, people were convinced that drinking must be to blame. In relation to the word 'dishevelment', it was later confirmed that PSP was active, and proves my point that some people wrongly connected his condition to alcohol.

Likewise, Dudley Moore also carried the burden of these types of accusations. He had been reported as being drunk, or friends and fans mistook him for his Arthur character when his illness first caused his speech to slur. It was said that he'd lost work, and rumours spread that he had a drinking problem.

In truth, Cilla was the only one of these known to have an alcohol problem and, therefore, given this evidence, I have come to the conclusion that PSP is not alcohol related. I could be wrong, and if I am proved wrong then I will be glad, since this mere declaration would prove that PSP has gained some form of progress in finding out its very cause.

If anything, I would like to point out the numerous amount of epidurals Cilla endured, and would think this is more likely to be a consideration than alcohol.

Once more, I would like to remind you that Cilla knew this subject was going to be on the agenda, but she did not mind... Her unequivocal response: *'Tell them!'*

2002

On the 22nd of August, Cilla was sent to have a esophagogastroduodenoscopy (EGD), which is a diagnostic endoscopic procedure that visualises the upper part of the gastrointestinal tract up to the duodenum. This is considered a minimally invasive procedure since, as such, it does not require an operation into any of the major body cavities. Nor does it require any significant recovery time after the procedure unless sedation or anaesthesia has been used in the process.

Due to the nature of the technique, a sore throat is common afterwards, and this affected Cilla because, for once, she temporarily fell silent. This was a useful investigative route, since it eliminated several considered problems Cilla was thought to be suffering from at the time.

Finally, in September, Cilla was diagnoses with gallstones. To deal with this, an endoscopic cholecystectomy was performed to surgically remove the gallbladder.

This is a widespread remedy of dealing with symptomatic gallstones.

Her recovery time was remarkably quick, and the symptoms she had been experiencing up and until then disappeared soon after.

2003

With all that had gone on in Cilla's life, I am not surprised she was eventually diagnosed with depression. However, she fought this opinion since she was convinced she did not have the illness. Furthermore, she disputed the findings and was convinced that there was more to this and tried, extremely hard, to prove otherwise. Sure, there were elements that on paper appeared to be depression, but somehow this seemed wrong to her. She even convinced me to look beyond the diagnosis and see what we could find. Living with Cilla meant I understood her better than anybody else, and fully understood what she meant. We probed deeper, but got no further than suggesting that her daily medication was wrong, so we pursued this direction further. Following a mere change in prescription, Cilla appeared to be more relaxed and started to cope better in any given situation.

From my perspective, and with hindsight, I am still wondering if the foundations of PSP were being laid out before us.

2005

December 2005 saw Cilla complaining of repeated trips to the toilet to urinate. You must understand that when I use the word complaining, I do not mean that in its truest sense. What I actually mean is that she often mentioned it without the emphasis on the word complaining, or what it actually implies.

This often interfered with her nightly sleep patterns, and whenever we went out she always made sure toilets were readily available. Eventually she sought help and was diagnosed with frequency of micturition. Under normal circumstances, the need to urinate is under voluntary control. However, in infants, some elderly, and those with neurological injuries, urination may occur as a reflex instead. Usually, adults tend to urinate up to seven times during the day, but in Cilla's case this was much more often.

Following several doctor's appointments, we found that there was only one solution.

Now here is the science bit: technically, by inserting a tube into the urethra, the capacity of the bladder when full can then be measured. Following this, the bladder is then gently stretched with fluid whilst under slight pressure to increase its capacity.

This initially helped, and Cilla's need to pee waned accordingly, however, this predicament would present itself again later, but as a much larger problem.

2009

Although not a direct medical issue, the following event may well have been connected to Cilla's final diagnosis. Also, for me, there were subsequent health related concerns, so I think it fair to mention the implications of this incident in this section of the overall story.

Cilla took a well-earned rest by driving to St Ives to be with Joe and his family, whilst I represented us both at a friend's wedding. The date was the 25th of April, and the distance between us at the time was as far apart as the weather was. Where I was, in Basingstoke, the temperatures were in their high seventies, with cloudless skies and intense sunshine, whilst in St Ives, there were much lower temperatures, equally low clouds and drizzle.

The bride, Sabrina, had just entered the room and the music started to play as David, the groom, took a nervous look back towards his bride-to-be. As this romantic interlude took place, my phone started to vibrate. Under the circumstances I would normally have left it, but something made me look at the screen, which clearly had the name 'CILLA' displayed upon it. Stealthily I crept out of the room and into the foyer before ringing her back because the phone had stopped vibrating before I could leave the room.

Cilla was very matter of fact, saying, *'I've had an accident.'*

My mind went into overdrive, especially since the distance between us was 234 miles, and I felt completely helpless on hearing this. I asked if she was hurt, but her only two concerns were for our 'Schnoodle' (Schnauzer Poodle cross) Charlie, who was in the car with her, and getting on with her journey.

She finally convinced me she was well and said, *'If somebody could just pull the wing out then I can get on my way. I don't think anything too serious is wrong with the car. Poor Charlie flew off the seat. I hit a hedge with a small wall behind it.'*

From where I stood, I had to make all of the arrangements with the insurance company and breakdown services. I eventually phoned Cilla back and asked her to call me as soon as the breakdown man arrived, so I could speak to him to assess my next move. From my anxious perspective, the return phone call took far too long to arrive, but eventually it did.

I spoke to the breakdown man who, in his ultimate wisdom and professional opinion, told me, *'The car's buggered, mate... I would say it's a write-off.'*

He handed the phone back to Cilla... I first explained the situation to her then arranged for her to be taken back to Joe's house before I finally went back to the ceremony.

Armed with the knowledge that the damaged car was now on the back of a low loader and on its way back to Hampshire, and in the early hours of the following morning, I set off to St Ives to collect Cilla. On arrival, Cilla showed me the bruising to her chest, stomach and right shoulder where the seat belt had fortunately snapped into position. I now realise that with the airbags failing to deploy, her injuries could have been much worse if the angle of impact had been more acute. Indeed, this also told me that the impact speed had been greater than Cilla had first led me to believe. She told me that apart from a wet road, she did not know how it had happened, and was still convinced the damage had not been as great as the breakdown man had suggested. It was not until five days later when I went to collect all of the belongings from the damaged car, that I realised just how much damage had occurred... and believe me, it was extensive.

Ironically, the car had been taken to a holding yard less than one mile from where I was when the drama started to unfold.

Importantly this event in Cilla's life meant that the outward trip to Cornwall, and the short trip prior to the accident, was the last time Cilla drove a car. To Cilla, and a lot of us, driving is a form of freedom, and to take that ability away meant restrictions and confinement.

Crucially though, this was not Cilla's last trip to St Ives.

On the night/early hours of the morning of the 15th of April 2016, and as close to the hour of her death, I took her remaining ashes there as per her request. I say remaining; because the rest were interred closer to home, where I frequently visit. Anyhow, from a high vantage point and on a moonlit night, with uncompromising passion, her ashes were 'liberated' into a strong prevailing wind. From my perspective, her ashes appeared to hover for a second or two, before swirling around and soaring off towards the sea. It was almost as if she was getting her bearings before setting off on this final journey.

For a split second or two, I felt totally exhilarated as I watched from both within the space I was occupying, and then from beyond the seascape before she finally disappeared.

Nobody else witnessed this scene, but I can tell you, it was extraordinarily breath-taking.

Although very personal, I really wanted you all to share in this moment!

Anyhow, it is only now that we enter the realms and outer boundaries of PSP.

It is a known fact that people who are eventually identified with PSP can go for years without true diagnosis due to the complexities of the illness... this was certainly true in Cilla's case.

On the 30th of September 2009, Cilla attended an appointment with a group in Southampton directly linked with the ME Association. The group mainly dealt with the phenomenon once termed as 'yuppie flu', or to give it its correct title: chronic fatigue syndrome (CFS) or myalgic encephalopathy (ME). Without complicating things further, CFS and ME are one and the same.

If I wanted to complicate matters, then I could have introduced three other acronyms for the disorder, which would have been somewhat confusing.

Anyhow, this is a complex medical condition, characterised by long-term fatigue and other related symptoms. These symptoms generally limit a person's ability to carry out day-to-day activities, and largely the life of a person with CFS or ME is usually and extremely compromised.

Anyhow, back to the appointment.

For some unknown reason, I was excluded from all of the sessions Cilla took part in, although I had to be there because I was, by now, her only means of transport.

Incidentally, Cilla had requested my presence during the sessions since she felt uncomfortable without me being within sight, but she was declined this wish.

As I waited in the reception area, I met several people – all women – awaiting their appointments. During the first visit, I never took much notice, and occupied myself by reading until Cilla returned. On the second visit, and partly out of boredom, I asked two of the attendees if they thought their ongoing visits were worthwhile. I did this because I had hope, thinking that these were the successes of the programme, but was amazed to find out that this was their first visit. This revelation made me think about the original opinion that Cilla had CFS/ME, because I could see no correlation between them and Cilla. Here were two women who, outwardly, could do all the things Cilla could not. Of course, their plight was genuine, but from a laypersons point of view, I knew Cilla's condition was somewhat different.

To highlight this point, I have included an extract from a letter written to Cilla's doctor and cc'd to her, dated the 15th of October and following her visits:

'It was difficult to make a definitive diagnosis of *Chronic Fatigue Syndrome/ME on Mrs Dagnell due to her very low mood and the fact that at present she has very little motivation due to this. Her score on the HADS scale today were 17 out of 21 for depression and 7 out of 21 for anxiety. She feels her depression is different to the depression she has experienced in the past in that she also has significant fatigue, joint pain in her back, neck and knees, waking up during the night, unrefreshing sleep, <u>slurred speech</u>, <u>frequent falls</u> and her <u>handwriting has become illegible</u>. I understand she has had a brain scan from her neurologist, which showed no abnormalities. There was concern about her memory and we did a Mini Mental State Examination (MMSE) on her in the clinic for which she scored 28 out of 30, comfortably within the normal range.'*

Firstly, I am convinced Cilla's scores on the HADS test and the score relating to anxiety were due to the fact that she felt under pressure, and almost certainly because I was not allowed to accompany her. Secondly, and perhaps more importantly, there were three noticeable and extremely significant points in that letter to which I have underlined. Knowing what I know now, I found this analysis to be quite revealing in the eventual diagnosis of PSP. Of course, this is not conclusive, but in my humble opinion it should have been considered at the time, or at least followed up as a possibility.

Once discharged from the clinic, Cilla attended several psychotherapy sessions, which she said she found both degrading and unhelpful. She also said she knew there was no need for her to see a psychologist but felt compelled to follow orders in the hopes she would eventually discover what was wrong with her.

Following a recent discovery, I found that Cilla actually disputed several points raised in these sessions. The discovery in question was an email to a friend, which challenged some of the findings that were written in the report to her doctor.

Reality Check

F aintly I hear you ask: Was it absolutely necessary for me to tell you all about Cilla's life in such detail up and until now?

To be frank, yes it was. In fact, I would go one stage further and say that it was absolutely imperative that you got to know the person... through good and bad!

Indeed, it is most important for you to realise that I am talking about a real individual here, and despite some very interesting aspects in her life, she was just like you and me: we are, without doubt, all similar in thought, hopes, dreams and aspirations.

Furthermore, by now you have also learnt that Cilla was a giving, passionate, active, go-getting, do it now sort of person. 'Live for the day' appeared to be one of her living and breathing mottos. And yes, undoubtedly you have discovered that she was active – sometimes well beyond human endurance. Cilla was one of those people who, when knocked down, would immediately get up, dust herself down, and do it all again.

Without doubt, when I look back for the first time since I met Cilla, I realise that her medical life was absolutely peppered with problems. Only now have I also had the opportunity of studying her health issues first-hand, despite living through it with her on a daily basis. Over the years, each condition was dealt with and due to time constraints appeared to virtually dissolve into one of life's little dramas.

I suppose the way we live our lives today, and with the pace of life as it is, we often forget the ailments, large and small, that others experience. If somebody suffers from cancer, we tend to roll the entire illness into one and treat it as a whole, whereas the sufferer lives with being subjected to day-to-day pain and endured anxiety.

In Cilla's instance, she complained little and, more importantly, never dwelt on her own pain or discomfort.

It is amazing to think that many of the people mentioned in the front of the book... and please take time to read their names... only knew Cilla during her darkest moments; yet, each and every one of them fell in love with the person she was. Most, if not all, openly wished that they had known Cilla in better days. In general, their views were echoed and mirrored throughout her life, since people just wanted to be part of her, purely in the hopes their lives would become enriched and as much fun as hers appeared to be. The saying, 'If I could bottle it, I would make a fortune' comes to mind.

Undeniably, what makes this story even more special is that communication, as part of Cilla's daily life, was not only essential but fashioned her very career. Being the hub of attention at work, especially in the reception area, meant she needed to be adept at communicating at the highest level. As you have read so far, even socially she needed those self-same skills to communicate on all levels within society. From Lords to paupers, she enticed, enthralled and captivated them all with the power of her communicative dexterity.

This is why she did not just want to tell you how we coped with the illness – anybody in a comparable position could have done that – no, what she wanted to do here is develop an understanding that we are all linked by one very exacting fact: mortality!

Cilla came into this world just like you or me, so where is the difference? Of course, many people develop illnesses that will eventually take their lives... again, where is the difference? The difference is not as immediate or as apparent as one might suspect, so I need you to read on and see how we managed from day one of Cilla developing PSP, and how and when we realised there was a problem and so on.

To do this, I shall highlight each subject in some form of order.

2010

From June and for a few months after, Cilla had several appointments which involved both scans and hip injections. Ironically, these appointments and procedures were conducted in Hythe, one of her old stomping grounds. This locational connection directly linked her to her past, and was the only pleasure Cilla received out of our visits there. I am convinced she would have been quite happy just to have visited the New Forest purely for pleasure, and not gone through the trials and tribulations of the various hospital appointments.

By now Cilla could not get around easily without the use of a wheelchair, which to her seemed so out of character and almost bordering on defeatism. She loathed being denied the ability to walk properly.

But this was just the start of things to come...

In the latter days of August, and thanks to Dr Olivia Rodrigues, our GP, Cilla was advised to see a Parkinson's specialist in Winchester. Believe it or not, Cilla actually smiled when it was suggested that she might have Parkinson's. This was not a happy smile, but a smile of liberation... in reality, it was a relief to be able to understand that there was a genuine reason behind all the suffering and indignity of being pushed around in a wheelchair.

The appointment was set and we appeared far too eager by misjudging the traffic and arriving an hour early. Patiently we sat in the local coffee house and awaited the allotted appointment time. We chatted about nothing in particular as the hour seemed to drag on longer than any before it.

Although we did not know it at the time, the importance of this appointment eventually became apparent to the both of us since a true diagnosis was now close at hand.

Dr Pinto was prompt, quiet and fully understanding of Cilla's plight. Although tacit, he sensed more than we appreciated; but he could not be sure without conducting specific secondary tests. Certainly, if he suspected PSP in the first instance – and I am convinced he did – then he kept it to himself. Even at this stage we were unaware of the term PSP, but under the circumstances, why should have we been? By now it was November, and on reviewing Cilla's earlier MRI scans and noticing that they were 'normal', he proposed one more. This time, he arranged a DaTSCAN.

A DaTSCAN is, I understand, a more complex imaging technique than the MRI scan. It uses small amounts of a radioactive drug to help determine how much dopamine is available in a person's brain. The device is similar to the MRI machine but smaller and is sometimes called a single-photon emission computed tomography – or SPECT scanner. Expertly, it measures the amount and location of the dopamine in the brain.

In itself, a DaTSCAN cannot alone diagnose Parkinson's disease; however, there are several other diseases – like progressive supranuclear palsy (PSP) – which also exhibits a loss of dopamine in the brain. It is because of this that the scans are often used to help a doctor confirm a diagnosis. In essence, the results of a DaTSCAN can be used to help rule out other diseases that may have similar characteristics and symptoms. However, largely, the DaTSCAN cannot alone differentiate between any other diseases and Parkinson's.

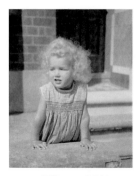
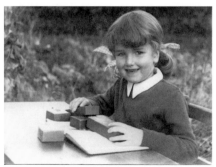

Cilla aged 2½
1951

Cilla's first day at school
1954

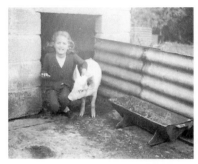
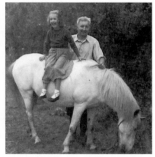

Cilla with Sally the Pig
Little Timbers

Cilla with her Father
Douglas & Poppet Circa
1957

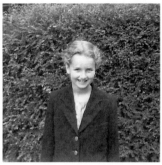

Cilla Circa 1960

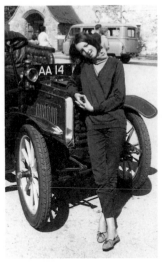

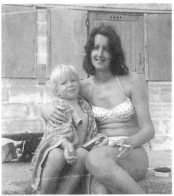

*Cilla outside the Domus
Beaulieu Standing in front of
the 1903 Panhard-Levassor*

*Cilla & her Son Joe
Circa 1973*

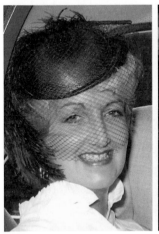

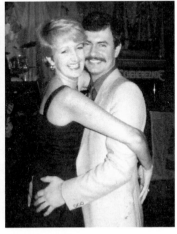

*Cilla Wedding Day
16.09.1982*

*Cilla & Steve
ACLS Function 1982*

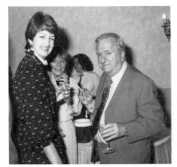

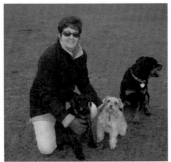

Cilla with Hugh Lloyd & his wife Shan, Sheraton Park Hotel London 11.10.1984

Cilla with Charlie, Bubbles & Ruby, Royal Victoria Country Park January 2006

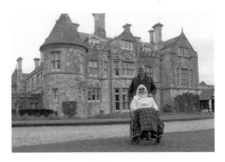

Cilla & Steve during her final visit to her beloved Palace House 07.05.2012

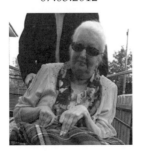

Cilla 14.09.2015 on route to see Priscilla Queen of the Desert

Steve Dagnell

Technical Issues

However, on top of everything else, we had one more hurdle thrown our way – and this one was something we could not easily ignore.

What was about to happen next was an interruption of such importance to us that I cannot move on without mentioning it... especially since there were also medical issues involved.

Right in the middle of the aforementioned events, our property was found to have major structural problems. Almost every room in the house developed major cracks, some of massive proportions. I can clearly remember that, from the outside, Cilla could actually put her hand through several of the worst cracks and was able to touch mine from the other side. Repairs would eventually be extensive, and every room would need refurbishing once the ground, plaster and brickworks were completed.

Anyhow, after some wide-ranging to-ing and fro-ing, the two insurance companies involved decided to do the decent thing and temporarily move us out whilst urgent repairs were carried out. We eventually did move out and would be gone six months to the day of leaving. Oddly, and under the circumstances thankfully, our temporary accommodation was exactly five miles away and within sight of one of our previous houses. This helped us considerably, since we were not only familiar with the area but with many of the local residents. Also, both hospitals – Winchester and Southampton – were still within the catchment area, so any notes and records were readily available should they be needed.

Two notable things happened while we were there – one of them being potentially very serious and relates to something I mentioned earlier!

By now Cilla was having problems with slight urinary incontinence, and wore both pads and protective knickers. Rather than be embarrassed, this combination gave her confidence to move around as freely as she could under the circumstances. However, whilst trying for the bathroom one evening she fell beside her bed, and due to my own health restrictions, I was not in a position to help her back on her feet. Using a combination of dog leads tied to the bed's structure and more than enough encouragement from me, she finally got off the floor and back on the bed. In all, I think the whole episode lasted just over an hour. During her time there it was obvious that this issue would come up again, so we later talked about future solutions.

Understandably Cilla decided that, if given the option, she would rather be in bed than mobile. She was already using her wheelchair more frequently, and some of this lack of mobility went back to both her knee and back operations. The bed itself also proved to be a problem rather than a solution because it did not adequately support her, and the height of the bed was wrong for her tall stature. This seemed like an ideal time to make proper plans for our return back home, so I contacted the various departments within Social Services. Finally, it was both agreed and planned that by the time Cilla arrived home, a hospital bed would be in situ. The cooperation we received from Social Services from that day forth was, in one word: *extraordinary!*

Now for the potentially serious situation I had mentioned.

On the evening of the 12th of December, I had gone out for the evening and left Cilla comfortably in bed. At this time, she was still administering her own medication – providing I had prepared any packaging – and before I left I made sure she had taken all her medication, with the exception of her sleeping pills. In this instance, all I did was pop the childproof cap off and leave it balanced on the top. This was something I had done for months, and under normal circumstances, Cilla was extremely careful when it came to drugs.

On my return I immediately noticed two things: firstly, the table top next to the bed was a total mess, and most of the items were either on their sides or on the floor; secondly, and more importantly, Cilla's breathing was quite shallow and she was resting in an unusual position. Up and until we moved back home, Cilla always slept on her stomach... and in this instance, she was not.

On closer examination, I noticed the top of the sleeping pill container was on the floor and the bottle itself was on its side... I then picked up the bottle. Strangely the bottle was empty, and there were no signs of the pills either on the table or on the floor. Furthermore, I noticed that it contained a residue similar to her mango juice. My mind quickly calculated the situation. Immediately I started shaking Cilla into consciousness with one hand, whilst dialling for an ambulance with the other. Although I was able to rouse her, and because of her now defective speech pattern, I could not make too much sense of her answers to my questions – by now, getting her off the bed and into a standing position was near on impossible.

Just before the ambulance arrived, I finally made some sense of what she was trying to tell me. Apparently, what had happened was that she had knocked her drink over, which in turn toppled the cap off the pill box and it filled up with the excess liquid. She did her best in clearing up the ensuing mess, but without thinking she drank the pill box full of mango juice because she did not want to waste any of the liquid; the thought had never crossed Cilla's mind that the now dissolved pills were harmful, or that she had actually consumed every pill in there.

A quick calculation on my part told me that Cilla had just consumed eighteen tablets in one go. Fortunately, in this instance, the tablets in question were the less harmful 7.5 milligram Zopiclone.

I must reiterate this point for any doubters that Cilla had no intention of harming herself, and had shown both concern and fear by the time of realisation.

The ambulance arrived and soon we were both being transported to the hospital. The doctors were quick to respond, and due to other issues, immediately started Cilla on a course of Trimethoprim for a previously undetected UTI, which might well have been influential in her confusion at the time.

Of course, the doctors asked all the pertinent questions, and after taking great care in sensitively talking to Cilla and carefully listening to her responses, came to the right and sensible conclusion.

During the night, my son Adrian, Cilla's brother Paul and his wife Jill, joined me at the hospital for support. This would be the first of many sleepless nights we would get throughout Cilla's illness.

Following a review from the hospital's RRT (Rapid Response Team), she was discharged and returned home none the worse for wear. Once out of hospital, Cilla did acknowledge concern over her actions and further restated her anxieties for what had happened. As a result of this, a plan was then put in place to prevent this type of accident from happening again.

Now imagine if Cilla had been living alone during this worrying time, and a family member had unsuccessfully tried to reach her and lived too far away to help. Or a neighbour was concerned that they had not seen her for a day or so. Perhaps in this scenario, Cilla had been struggling on the floor and unable to get up... ? I shuddered to think of the answers, but it did highlight various issues.

Due to this concern, this is a particularly good time to express a point about a scheme that has already helped save countless lives. It is so simple in its design, that I am surprised I had not heard about it any sooner.

At the time of this incidence, my son Adrian was a first responder for the South Central Ambulance Service and told me about a charity based scheme known as *Lions Message in a Bottle*.

Firstly, let me explain something about first responders. These are highly trained professional people who work alongside ambulance crews and clinically qualified practitioners. To maximise their effectiveness, they are directly linked to the ambulance network via telephone, and are called in any medical emergency situation within their own area. Invariably, they are the first person to arrive on the scene ahead of either a paramedic or an ambulance crew... thus the title, first responder. Within their lifesaving capacity, they carry essential apparatus such as heart monitoring equipment and defibrillators, along with the skills to use them. Usually, they live within a limited distance from any potential patient, hence their ability to arrive so quickly on a scene. Likewise, whilst in their day-to-day civilian life they are always available, and often put themselves forward in any given medical situation or emergency. Indeed, many people today owe their lives to these unsung heroes.

Anyhow, Lions Message in a Bottle simply tells any member of the emergency services that a person living at a particular address has a health issue. Simply put, a tightly capped, green and white plastic bottle containing medical details of the patient or sufferer of a life threatening illness is placed in their fridge. To accompany this, a recognised sticker is placed on the front door which triggers the actions of any emergency responder from any of the three major services. Their immediate course of action would be to obtain the bottle on entry. Of course, the availability of a key safe would also assist in this matter.

Even if the patient is unconscious, the responder can read the content and very quickly ascertain up to date medical history thus saving valuable time. BUT, it is up to the day-to-day carers to keep this information up to date... especially where medication is concerned!

The bottle is large enough to contain several folded A4 sheets of paper, which could include a DNR (do not resuscitate) order or DNACPR (do not attempt cardio pulmonary resuscitation) directive and, as already indicated, should also list medications.

From their website –
http://lionsclubs.co/Public/lions-message-in-a-bottle/
– I was able to glean the following:

'More than 5 million FREE Message in a Bottle kits have been distributed by Lions Clubs British Isles & Ireland in recent years to people with conditions such as diabetes, allergies, disabilities and life-threatening illnesses.

The bottles are supplied FREE of charge thanks to generous donations from the public and businesses.

Lions clubs supply the bottles to health centres, doctors' surgeries and chemists. They are also available direct from Lions clubs – contact us for more information.

Paramedics, police, fire-fighters and social services support this life-saving initiative and know to look in the fridge when they see the Lions Message in a Bottle stickers.'

As you can see, apart from the three major emergency services, Social Services also support this initiative, and I urge you to include this in your arsenal in battling against PSP.

Cilla's 50th Birthday, 1999

N ow, in true time warp fashion, I am going to take you back to a story I had alluded to earlier, and have placed it here so I did not upset the balance regarding Cilla's medically related history.

This venture revolved around a genuine milestone in Cilla's life, and one she wanted to celebrate in style... so her first mistake was to leave it up to me to organise it! In fact, it did not turn out to be too bad after all, since I decided on a cruise. Yes... that is what she thought too... until I told her it was going to be on The Thames with friends.

Since the decision was originally made in May 1998, I had just over a year to organise the trip, and came up with a plan to finance it in such a way that it would be easier on the pocket for all concerned. I asked each friend to contribute a £30 deposit and £5 a month thereafter, which would be banked in a high interest account.

Apart from myself, there was only one other man involved – Eilef, who is the husband of Sue Loken, and a long-time friend of Cilla's. Excluding Cilla and the previously mentioned, the rest of the crew consisted of Barbara Avery, Isobel Howard, Ann Weakley, Sue Donaldson and Beverley Oakes (Allan) – again, all very close friends of Cilla's.

Although Cilla's birthday was not until July, the most convenient date for all concerned was from Saturday the 19th of June 1999, and for one week.

To get the best out of this week's holiday, we decided to meet up in Windsor the night before and stay in a hotel. The timing could not have been better, since I booked the Clarence Hotel – situated in the heart of Windsor – one year in advance without the knowledge of a coinciding royal wedding! Fortunately for us, it was not until the 6th of January 1999 that Prince Edward announced his engagement to Sophie Rhys-Jones, now the Countess of Wessex.

As I have already said, our timing could not have been better, since the wedding was also to take place on the 19th of June 1999 at St George's Chapel, Windsor Castle. Had we left our hotel booking till January or beyond, then it would have been impossible for us to find accommodation for the preceding night. Furthermore, I am convinced that hotel prices in the area would have escalated exponentially on the announcement of their engagement!

To enhance the event, I hired a Sony DCR-TRV103 Digital8 camcorder, which was both substantial in size compared to today's standard, and a totally new experience for us all.

Given the preparations, the only thing I could not arrange was the weather, which under the circumstances proved to be quite good after a bad start! And ironically, it was Beverley who had an actual birthday on-board, which was another pure but happy coincidence.

Talking of coincidences, not knowing that they were already friends, I had actually met Beverley about one year before I actually knew Cilla. In this instance Beverley worked for a rival shipping line based in Southampton and was yet another one of my *Southern Evening Echo* customers.

Anyhow, my forward projection regarding finances paid off, since we were able to pay for everything from the savings account I had set up for this specific event. Indeed, once the Clarence Hotel in Windsor, hire of the boat, fuel, water, mooring fees and septic tank waste fees were taken into account, we had enough left to pay for a first nights feast in a local Italian restaurant.

This turned out to be a momentous trip and one we all remember to this day... although some for the wrong reasons! To be fair, the occurrence I am referring to did not transpire until after we arrived back at the boatyard, where Sue Donaldson found that her car had been stolen. With Isobel and their luggage in tow, I persuaded a reluctant yard manager to drive them the seventy-odd miles home.

Incidentally, her car was eventually found burnt out in Essex, and following an involvement in a post office robbery.

Even to this day, I am able to snuggle down and quite literally look back on those heady days due to the fact I transferred the video tape of the trip onto disc. Once more, this shows how important visual memories are, because one main overriding feature of the disc is still being able to listen to Cilla both talk and laugh!

& PSP

2011

In sequence, during Cilla's next appointment with Dr Pinto, and following the results of the DaTSCAN, the acronym PSP appeared to conspire against her. To be fair, Dr Pinto was at his gentlemanly best, but knowing what I know now, we were about to take the first steps into Cilla's preordained future.

On this significant day in Cilla's life, Wednesday the 26th of January 2011, we first heard of, or officially had any concept or connection with the term PSP. Already, Dr Pinto was finally convinced that Cilla was not suffering from Parkinson's and told Cilla he was going to ask a colleague of his to see her.

Dr Pinto carefully explained the difference between the two illnesses, but in truth, I think it was far too early for us to realise the full impact.

Similarly, as was the case when Cilla was told that she had ME and Parkinson's, there was a certain amount of relief knowing she was finally being acknowledged as a sufferer of a particular illness. She also hoped that this would be the last diagnosis, without fully realising the full impact PSP would have on her life. This is a point, I think, that all PSP sufferers have to go through before finally being recognised as a genuine patient. Likewise, at the time, to us there seemed less significance on the implications of the illness than the final diagnosis... but that would soon change.

On the 26th of June, we had our first appointment with Dr Manson, a colleague of Dr Pinto's and also based in Winchester. Dr Manson specialises in movement disorders and, like Dr Pinto, is also a consultant neurologist. Equally, they share knowledge of Parkinson's, but Dr Manson mainly deals with the rarer subject of PSP.

From here we would finally learn more about the horrors of PSP... although this was done with utmost sympathy and sincerity. The disorder was fully explained to us and each stage mapped out, for which we were extremely grateful.

As far as the symptoms were concerned, everything now slotted into place and, given the final verdict, we could finally see how Cilla's condition corresponded to her immediate physical state. It all added up: the instantaneous and impromptu backward falls, the stuttering and the handwriting... everything now made sense!

We now had all the factors in place to formulate a plan of action – although Cilla was yet to have one more conclusive test, which I shall address later.

For now, we studied everything we could about the condition, and by bypassing Internet references to Sony's Play Station Portable – PSP! – we were finally able to conduct a feasible and constructive strategy.

Once we knew what the diagnosis was, I asked Cilla what our plan of action should be. As usual she surprised me with her answer, which was simple but emphatic by saying: '*Let people know!*'

To emphasise her wishes, I started taking notes during our various discussions, and these summaries certainly helped later, since I was able to capture specific moments in time. Mostly, these notes were taken over a short period of time, since we eventually decided to keep a blog. In conjunction with this, I continued to write and kept taking useful notes throughout Cilla's illness, hence the ability to now follow her progress and definitively present the findings right up to her last moments.

The sole intention of the blog was to help others understand both the illness and how it affects the person involved. Indeed, every carer who ever had an input into Cilla's daily care, was asked to read her blog so they fully understood her dilemma. Once again, this was Cilla's way of preparing for the future.

In the meanwhile, and fortunately, Cilla was still able to type, which allowed me to understand her better since her speech was now getting more and more slurred – although typing too would finally lose its effectiveness.

Some elements of what you are about to read are a repeat of what I have already said, but importantly, these are Cilla's words. Also, you must realise that her words took more time than usual to create and type, since her abilities to sit for any length of time was already compromised, as was her sight.

Her thoughts are as follows:

'Like everybody, we sometimes rely on lists. In this instance, I remember going to a supermarket and wondering what the scrawl was I had written down as a shopping list. This particular list was as difficult for me to read as it was for others. Over the coming months, trying to decipher what I had written became more of a problem as time went by. Eventually, my husband Steve had to take over writing cards on my behalf. In truth, it was first deemed a bit of a joke, but as time went on it became worrying since other signs started to come to the fore.

Take my eyesight as an example: here I became more prone to bright light than ever. By this I mean, even in the dullest of days I felt the need to wear sunglasses whenever I went out. Apart from the occasional odd look from strangers, I felt comfortable wearing the glasses and wore them out every time I left the house.

Overriding all of the first few symptoms was my lethargy and tiredness. I felt tired for no apparent reason and felt more comfortable in bed. Here I could sleep. However, even after a good sleep I felt just as tired. This affected my daily life and things started to become less important around me. I did not neglect housework or anything like that; no, I just found everything harder to do. Sometimes, just getting out of bed was an effort, so it seemed easier to stay!

After a while, I felt that the situation was becoming ridiculous, so I made an appointment with a doctor. The doctor examined me, and quickly came to the conclusion that I had ME. Commonly known as yuppie flu, it is in fact chronic fatigue syndrome &/or myalgic encephalomyelitis.

Following an online search, I suppose I cannot really blame the medical profession for that diagnosis since these are the symptoms of ME: debilitating low energy levels, painful muscles and joints, disordered sleep, gastric disturbances, poor memory and concentration, neuropsychological complaints, painful lymph nodes and prolonged fatigue after exercise.

But subconsciously I knew there was something missing from the equation, although I did nothing to question it.

Anyhow, having what I thought was ME somewhat helped my state of mind, since my condition had been going on for far too long. Giving the ailment a name was rather comforting, since it meant I was not making it all up. I am still convinced there were a few people who could not understand the predicament I now found myself. Anyhow, I had some form of respite due to this revelation.

As time progressed two things happened, both of them at the behest of my doctor. Firstly, I was assigned a psychologist, since the events over the years had taken its toll and I was deemed depressed. Secondly, I had an appointment to be examined by a professional within the ME Association. The most important of the two, in my mind, was the visits to the ME Association's centre based close to where I live. What made these visits important was that my husband made an observation and asked me to give an opinion. This I did and casually observed other 'patients' and soon came to my own conclusion. Seeing them arrive, pick up a magazine, read for a while, then freely move into their appointment made me wonder. I wondered if they were the success stories and were there for their final follow-up appointments. As it happens, my husband found out that they were, in some cases like me, first or second time visitors. My final conclusion was that there were several levels and I must have been at the top of the tree!

Then something happened to make me look at everything again!

I was suffering from hot flushes and wanted to speak to a doctor about my medication for HRT. Hormone replacement therapy is something I saw as separate from my 'condition' and wanted to seek out better medication. Since my regular doctor was not available, I accepted an alternative appointment with a different doctor.

I dutifully attended the practice and, although stuttering, was able to tell the doctor everything that had happened over the last four years. She listened, showed concern and compassion, before referring me to see a specialist.

That was just over a year ago and I have now been catapulted into another dimension.

Over those years, my speech to some became somewhat alien. It appeared slurred and I even found myself being repetitive with single words. Soon, this became whole sentences and I found some of the people I was talking to were trying to help me finish what I was trying to say. You see, I knew exactly what I wanted to say but found it had been lost after it had left my brain. Somewhere between my brain and my mouth the words had sort of gotten jumbled up and did not come out as I had intended.

This somewhat inhibited my ability to be around people. Those that have known me from years ago have, in the past, found me sociable and, dare I say, an extrovert. I feel that this is an important point since it is how I was generally known. It made me... me!

I have already used the word alien... in that sense I was talking about my speech and myself. What happened next made me feel even more like an alien! Many people I had been in constant touch with started to fade into the background. Whether they found it difficult to understand me or whether it was me shying away from them, I do not know. Bit by bit they dwindled away and left us to it. I must admit in some respects this was a blessing, since it left me with less of a need to explain myself, which of course was already difficult.

In some respects, with fewer people in my life it became easier to get on with what was happening around me.

Coupled with the regular falls came the inevitable injuries. These mostly resulted in bruising, sometimes quite severe. What is strange

*about this is in the way I fall! Never forward...
always back! I have been seen doing it, and by all
accounts, I just 'go' without the capacity of self-
restraint. By that, I mean I am somehow unable to
put my arms or hands out to brace for impact or
prevent it from happening.*

*On one occasion I hit my head so badly I
needed medical assistance and an ambulance was
called. Five hours in A & E and several stitches
later, I was home. The strange thing here though
was the reaction of the nursing staff at the
hospital. Initially my wound was not even looked
at, and the emphasis seemed to centre on how I
came to fall. It was only in the last ten minutes of
my stay at A & E that my injury was looked at.
By then my hair was so matted with blood I had
to have some of my hair cut off so they could view
the wound.*

*I am convinced that the staff thought there was
an element of spousal abuse at work! You see,
there are many people in the health profession who
do not know about, or understand PSP! Indeed,
some have never even heard of it or, therefore, its
symptoms! The reason I mention this is to show
how difficult it is to convey what had happened. If
I'd had the full power of speech, then it would be
easy to answer some of the questions. Because I*

was slow and because of their lack of understanding, it was then left to my husband to explain what had happened. Even when he mentioned PSP, he received blank looks and more than a certain amount of incredulity. Suspicion was purely based on my inability to immediately answer their questions. I sheepishly looked at my husband for support, and am convinced it looked like I was looking for 'permission' to speak. Indeed, I desperately needed my husband to convey my version of accounts, simply because I could not. Their misinterpretation of the situation delayed my eventual treatment. Despite this, I fully understand the need to protect people in spousal abuse situations and wish for those suffering to remain strong.

There have been many more falls since then and I only really feel safe when I am in bed. There have also been more hospital visits... and more stitches. In some respects, I am lucky since I have taken to wearing a padded rugby-style helmet. This, although unflattering to look at, has already saved my life. How? Simple! I fell so hard that even with the helmet on I ended up with a massive bruise to the back of my head. Without the helmet, I am convinced I would have died through severe head trauma!

Despite this, I have other issues which are now becoming more prominent. Just a couple of days ago I went to the hospital to see if I could have help with my vision. This followed a routine visit to the opticians, who tested my sight and then referred me back to my doctor. With a little anxiety and a certain amount of expectation, the appointment date finally came. The problem with my sight is not just based on the light sensitivity; no, the problem is also rooted in occasional double vision and blurring. I soon found out that with PSP, some sufferers find relief after being fitted with prism lenses. From what I understand, the prisms allow the wearer to look at the world from another perspective. You see (no pun intended), I find it difficult to look up or down, which in my case also affects my balance. The prisms change one's perspective and, if successful, partly rights what the brain interprets.

Unfortunately, in my instance, after my eye test and testing with various lenses, it was deemed a failure. I was told by the specialist doctor, "Sorry, there is nothing we can do for you! You could try taping up one of your eyes, which would allow the brain to concentrate its efforts more efficiently."

So there you have it! Prisms will not help me, but some masking tape might! Still, we will give it a try. . .

For now, though, I have given you all enough to think about.'

By typing this out, Cilla found the exercise extremely therapeutic, although a chill runs down my spine when I now read Cilla's words... I suppose it reminds me of the times she could, in a fashion, talk and type and do certain things she would soon lose the ability to do.

Despite our newly acquired knowledge about the illness, I never for one minute suspected the illness would have such an impact on both of our lives.

The following is an exercise I used to track her handwriting abilities:

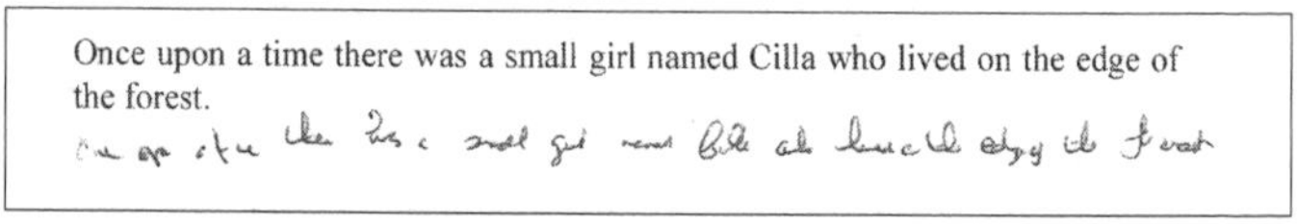
Once upon a time there was a small girl named Cilla who lived on the edge of the forest.

Although resembling a foreign language, this was Cilla's best efforts at the time.

Challenges

E arlier I mentioned one more conclusive test... a test Cilla was eager to take, and even more eager to hear about the outcome.

Bring on the DOPA challenge!

Prior to the test date, which was set for the 2nd of September 2011, Cilla was prescribed Domperidone 20mg TDS. Cilla was strictly required to take these for three days before the tests. This is quite significant and highly important to the success or failure of the test. I believe, although I could be wrong, the idea of the challenge is not to confirm PSP, but to disprove Parkinson's. By this I mean, should the test become positively conclusive due to the introduction of Dopamine to the system, and the symptoms improve accordingly, then Parkinson's is present.

Using this approach, it is possible to distinguish those patients who respond well to the medication. Likewise, if there is no improvement, then the alternative is a given – subject to the mental tests and the incorporation of some physical tests – and then it is *almost* (and I emphasis the word *'almost'* here with caution) certainly PSP.

These recommended tests were mostly employed to evaluate pre-surgical levels of depression and dementia. The tests also assess executive functions such as verbal fluency, immediate and delayed memory, reasoning ability, and shift in cognitive strategies.

In Cilla's case, she completed the tests, which included timed walks, selective finger movements, mini puzzles, drawing continual circles, eye movements, repetitive speech patterns and a few subtler experiments.

Following this, Cilla was given a measure of liquid – I suspect Dopamine again – and we were told we were free to have lunch or wander around for an hour or so.

This we did, and returned accordingly.

Unexpectedly the same sequence of tests were then repeated, once more against the clock. The final verdict, and now I could see the reasoning of repeating the tests, was that Cilla performed each set of tests in an almost identical time: in other words, the Dopamine had no effect or comparison.

In essence, PSP had *almost* been assured, and to be fair, by now I think Cilla and I had already accepted this conclusion.

The leading doctor in this case was Dr Boyd Ghosh, who asked if we could, for training purposes, authorise future use of the recordings they had taken – to which we both agreed. I actually retained a part-recording of that session myself, and often look back at that significant time in our lives together.

Remarkably, yet again, Cilla took control of the situation and started to make arrangements far beyond her eventual death. Her get-up-and-go spirit had once more emerged and she started to look at the future with renewed vigour.

Physical changes had already started to take place and her needs started to change accordingly. No longer was she able to do as much as she used to and, as you know, the only place she really felt both safe and comfortable was in bed.

Fortunately, the hospital bed was in place, and she could now rest at ease and not worry too much about falling – after a fashion she could get up and, within reason, do certain things.

Whilst on the subject of falls, you may recall that Cilla mentioned in her blog a padded rugby-style helmet. I bought this to prevent her from injuring herself after sustaining several head wounds following backward falls. The idea came to me when seeing the Czechoslovakian goalkeeper, Petr Čech, wearing the same style helmet. Čech, who sustained a head injury in 2006, underwent surgery for a depressed skull fracture and was initially unaware of the seriousness of the injury. The doctors looking after him later reported that the collision which caused the head injury nearly cost Čech his life.

In Cilla's instance, within a few days of me insisting she wear it every time she left the bed had a particularly nasty fall. As usual, she fell straight back and landed two steps below the height she was originally standing. I immediately rushed to her aid and finally got her up off the ground. On inspection she was badly bruised, but thankfully the helmet had done its job. Her scalp had sustained a large contusion, and I am convinced the fall would have killed her had she not been wearing the helmet.

Anyhow, going back to the previous subject, one of those things Cilla would leave her bed for was to visit the toilet.

Going to the loo so frequently was getting out of hand, and in some instances, despite the close proximity, the distance became too great. Already precautions were in place should there be the occasional 'accident', but these were becoming far too common. Okay, a quick change of pad and clean up was all that was required at the time, but ultimately this was not the problem. The problem was that her body did not recognise night from day, and these episodes were going on as much throughout the night as in the day, and to make matters worse, during the night and on several occasions Cilla would fall.

We sought further help, and as harsh as it sounds, the only suitable solution was a ureteral catheter. On the 16th of September, ironically our wedding anniversary, the district nurse turned up on our doorstep fully laden with equipment.

However, even this solution would initially cause various problems, but none more so than Cilla's tall stature, which immediately compromised the fitting. It quickly became apparent that the conventional female catheter was far too short in distance for the length of her legs, so a male alternative was inserted instead!

Immediately Cilla became more comfortable with the fit, and with the addition of night drainage bags we were able to create a better sleep pattern for us both. To assist further, Cilla wore her leg bag inside a specially designed footless 'sock', which firmly held the bag in situ and against her inner calf muscle. By changing this from leg to leg on a daily basis we reduced the risk of pressure sores. This method of care also avoided the need for her to wear the elasticated Velcro strip, commonly used to keep the bag and tube in place, and I am pleased to say that by using our method, Cilla never suffered sores – none whatsoever!

Of course it was essential that we keep an eye on proceedings, since having a permanent fitting can create its own little problems. On odd occasions, the urine would bypass the catheter due to blockages, so from a very early stage it was agreed that Cilla would continue wearing pads as a backup. There were also times when a small infection set in, and it was necessary to flush the system through using both the correct procedure and the necessary prescribed acidic fluids.

Providing the carers kept an eye on all aspects regarding the catheter, then I see no reason not to have one fitted... although in Cilla's case it was indispensable.

At the base of the leg bag is either a T-type valve or a lever tap-style valve, both designed for drainage. Below that is a short length of tubing which the urine is drained from. In our case, we always capped this off with the blue or grey disposable cap provided on all new units. This, in my opinion, served two purposes: firstly, with the cap covering this exit, any germs would be stopped from entering through that particular portal and, secondly, the cap is secured firmly enough to stop any leakages should the valve be accidently left open.

And, believe me, this can happen!

Since we made sure Cilla got up for each meal, the catheter bag was well looked after, and knowing what I know about the dynamics of water, I knew it was essential to keep an eye out for leaks and drips. Whilst in bed, a disposable waterproofed cotton-based mini-sheet was placed under Cilla's bottom and as high up as her lower back. The reason it was placed as high as it was, was because once again, the dynamics of water comes into effect, and I was always concerned that any possible leakage or blockage would cause further problems. The last thing I wanted was urine following the contours of the body and leaking upwardly and causing caustic burns to her back, or worse, continual bedsores.

Finally, two important points I found invaluable: the night bag was always hung on the base bar of the bed using the special hanger provided with the fresh supply of bags, and in turn, this was always hung over a washing up bowl to prevent any damage to the floor or carpet should there be any unfortunate accidental leakages.

Incidentally, the bottom section of the catheter containing the actual bag was changed when required, and the section leading into Cilla's urethra was always flushed through first. The catheter itself, and in its entirety, was changed by the district nurse on an eight-week cycle.

Communication

E ven though the majority of you have never actually met her, by now you know Cilla was usually very communicative, so her ever-diminishing powers of communication needed to be addressed.

This aspect needed to be sorted quickly since I, and others more so, found it difficult to understand Cilla's daily needs. In the early days, we used Cilla's remaining power of speech and plenty of patience to understand her, but as time went by, we needed an alternative. Using a conventional alphabet chart, we were more able to understand. It soon became obvious that the standard chart was lacking, so we developed our own to include the most important aspects of Cilla's day-to-day needs. Of course, we still had the complete alphabet, plus numbers one through to zero, which left us with fifteen blank boxes. Each blank space was then used to graphically highlight an emblem or easily recognised symbol. Looking at the chart before me now, I realise that given the space around the borders, we could have included nine more boxes if we so wished.

Anyhow, going through them we had the following graphics: a toothbrush, the sun, a person shivering, a sandwich, a catheter, a window, a toilet, a clock, a shower head, a bowl of cereal, a television remote control, a drink, earplugs, TV guide and a Rottweiler.

To some, this might be a strange combination, but to Cilla they represented most of what she needed, since the rest she could readily spell out. These shortcuts meant a quick point of the finger to the window icon would mean either open or close the window depending on its current position. Likewise, a person shivering or the sun would represent her personal temperature, which would need adjusting accordingly.

A Rottweiler? I hear you ask... Well, at that stage we still had one furry friend left but in May of 2012 we finally lost her too, so at the time, the graphic was purely there for Cilla to be reassured that I had walked or fed her that morning or afternoon.

No matter how we used the chart, others can always adapt to their own lifestyle and needs.

Of course, to use the chart it is necessary to summon somebody's attention, after all, it was not as if Cilla could call out. We did this by easily attaching a conventional bicycle bell to one of the dropdown side rails on the bed. Well within Cilla's reach, this became a very successful tool and, believe me, it was used extensively.

Even when this too became a problem for Cilla, I upgraded the system to a battery-operated remotely-linked doorbell. The small sender unit had no wires, so it was easily and neatly tucked into her pyjama top pocket. I had to be careful here because there were a few occasions when the remote control unit almost ended up in the washing machine!

In due course, the chart became ineffective due to Cilla's sight reducing to a degree that she could not identify either the symbols, alphabet or numbers. Fortunately, by now, we were able to foresee certain factors and had already devised a system of hand gestures and signs well before that eventuality became a reality. For instance, a forward facing clenched fist meant 'please check my catheter bag', likewise the palm inwards Winston Churchill style two-fingered salute pursed to her lips simply meant 'cigarette', or a horizontal flat hand with palm down meant 'bed controls'.

Once again, others can develop their own interpretation, but we soon learned one thing: it was always best and most productive, to ask Cilla a question that could simply be answered with a 'yes' or 'no' response. In those instances, the common response was either a thumbs-up for 'yes' or the vertically raised palm outward flat of the hand for 'no'.

When speech was completely out of the question, we had one other tool in our arsenal: invisible paper and pen. Here Cilla would use the flat of her left hand as paper and the index finger on her right hand to draw out a letter of the alphabet. This was also touch sensitive, so easier for Cilla to feel the letter too. Also, to save her time and energy, we adapted the fingers and thumb on the left hand as vowels, much like in the sign language Makaton. From the thumb to the little finger she could quite easily spell out A, E, I, O and U much quicker than the alternative use of the other twenty-one letters.

Obviously it is not as if we had invented the system, since one of the earliest written records of a sign language goes back to the fifth century BC.

In Plato's *Cratylus*, Socrates said: *'If we hadn't a voice or a tongue, and wanted to express things to one another, wouldn't we try to make signs by moving our hands, head, and the rest of our body, just as dumb people do at present?'*

To make this a more salient point, the Ethnologue, a commonly recognised and well-respected web-based publication, contains statistics for 7,469 languages and dialects. It also lists 137 uses of speech with signs, so in short, this method can be adapted to any country and culture in the world.

Once Cilla had completely lost the capacity to talk, I mourned and longed for those moments where we would talk for hours over mere trivia. However, and much to our surprise, every once in a while Cilla would speak! And although in this case the sentences were broken, the words were as clear as anything I had heard in our lifetime together.

I once took the opportunity to ask her about it in one of these rare and fleeting moments.

In this instance, I have picked up the conversation part way through:

Cilla – *'I'm speaking am I… am I?'*

Me – *'You're talking clearly.'*

Cilla – *'Am I? Am I?'*

Me – *'You are, yes.'*

Cilla – *'Gosh.'*

Me – *'As clear as day.'*

Cilla – *'Fancy that.'*

Me – *'Fancy that!'*

Cilla – *'I didn't… didn't… didn't know I was.'*

Me – *'You didn't know you were? Can you not hear yourself?'*

Cilla – *'No… '*

Me – *'No… ?'*

Cilla – *'I can hear buzz, buzz, buzz, buzz, buzz, buzzing in my ears.'*

Me – *'Buzzing in your ears… Can you hear anything?'*

Cilla – *'I can hear you… I can hear you.'*

This auspicious occasion sticks in my mind the most, and fortunately Georgie Huskins, who was also in the room, video recorded it all on her mobile phone. This and the other remaining part of the conversation all occurred on the 25th of March 2015 – although sadly, it only lasted for two minutes and thirty seconds. Alas, these occasions were extremely rare and there were only going to be a handful more of these short conversations left for us to treasure over the next nine months.

Before I continue, I wish to make a disclaimer, since my experience is purely based on what occurred in Cilla's life:

In no way should our experiences be taken as a valid reason for you to tear up the rule book. How you deal with your own illness or those affected by an illness should not be considered lightly or influenced by others. How you cope with the illness, or any other related illness during and beyond, must be discussed at length between yourselves as a family and your own medical practitioners.

For those carers who are reading this, or those of you who are in the very onset of PSP, I strongly suggest you arrange or, at least, do two things.

Firstly, and crucially, organise a plan of action regarding speech or a representative replacement for speech. Initially, plan together and when others are involved, bring them in on the plan. Certainly, do not leave this important issue too late.

And secondly, visually record as much of what you do when you can and while you can. Over all, this second point is sometimes less practical – although it can be used as a tool to teach others – but to me was much more important for the spouse and loved ones, since we were able to cherish these moments later.

Within the subject matter of communication, I now wish to include some practical advice about who to contact and what to do once diagnosed.

By now, any such fanciful idea about a cure has all but been lost and between the sufferer and the family, you have learnt one important fact: *you have sadly been given a death sentence.*

I cannot pretend to have enjoyed highlighting this point, but I think we are far enough into the book to drop any pretences about the final outcome. There now is a reason for me to be brutal, and not be meagre with the truth about the subject or about the eventual conclusion of this condition.

This stark, almost heartless caveat, is meant as a rally call to all parties involved... and I beg no forgiveness: *you must now be prepared.*

Remember, PSP will take much away from you in the initial stage, *but* it will never take away your powers of decision... providing you act quickly!

Be prepared to take the final pain and suffering away from the ones you leave behind. You must be practical about what is left of your life. Be realistic about your own final wishes... be like Cilla!

Cilla actually mapped out everything, from her funeral to well beyond. We frequently sat down at her behest and went through every detail of her funeral. To highlight this point, only four weeks prior to her own death we returned from a friend's funeral and Cilla asked me one more time to go through her order of service. It was during this session that she added one final piece of music to the order: *Beautiful Boy* by John Lennon.

The significance was purely hers and, I am certain, simply related to her son Joe. Once more she had shown the spirit that we would all like to display in the face of adversity, or in this case, death.

Nevertheless, even at the earliest point in time, I strongly suggest you do several things. For a start, make a will! This will not bring forth a sudden increase in your mortality... No! This will bring you nothing but peace of mind. If you have not already done so, get your finances in order and make sure nothing is left until the last minute.

Once you have made this, and before you do anything else, make another... this time I mean a living will, or sometimes known as a personal directive or advanced decision. This will outlines your wishes when you are no longer in a position to direct your own desires, needs and hopes. Later, you will find out how two of these made the difference to what Cilla actually wanted, and how they came about. No matter what the wish, put it down; but more importantly, concentrate on your medical needs and issues first.

By this I mean if you do not want to be resuscitated following some form of failure, then make that point clear. This can be added to all of your medical notes and will, by law, be observed if the right procedures are taken. The DNR (do not resuscitate), or DNACPR (do not attempt cardio pulmonary resuscitation), consideration is such an important aspect of how you are finally dealt with should the need arise.

This brings me to the first important point I made earlier when mentioning a living will. Cilla made this important choice on the 2nd of August 2012, and was gratefully taken into consideration on the 16th of December 2015, which finally eased her suffering. It is *vital* that you let people know what you want... after all, it is going to be your final decision!

Who else should you be in touch with?

Of course, contact any government departments that could help out with finances, such as the Department of Works and Pensions (DWP), since if you are not already receiving financial assistance then this would be the place to start.

There is, of course, your local council, which could offer further assistance in the form of a Social Worker. Most local government offices can put you through to the right department, probably Adult Social Care, so start there. Although already stretched, their resources can oblige you with a great deal of information, which includes important features such as Respite, Take a Break, care options and planning, nursing homes and a whole host of other details. Either way, explore them all... because, ultimately, you will need all the help you can get!

I mentioned Respite, which as a long term carer I found particularly useful... Unquestionably, and once again, I found it *vital!* Respite, in my case, allowed me up to the maximum of eight weeks a year to go away, or have the freedom to detach one's self from the daily routine. As selfish as this sounds, as a carer you often take on the illness as part of your daily routine. To be even more rudimentary in this assessment: the carer can walk away from the illness, unlike the sufferer. In some cases, it is extremely necessary to temporarily leave behind something others have to live with. Of course, there is no way you can forget what you have left behind, but if you do not take advantage of these opportunities, then you could end up becoming ineffectual at the very care the sufferer needs.

There is also another service some know little about: Take A Break. Unlike Respite, Take a Break offers the full carer a few hours a week to get away from the day-to-day events at home. In this time, you can either go shopping, take a short trip, visit friends and family, or anything else that takes your fancy.

Under these circumstances, a carer or family member could sit or take your place until you return, feeling refreshed and more willing to carry on. Conversely, where Respite is involved, it may be possible for the sufferer to spend a short stay in a nursing home, or have a carer or family member move in to the household. However, and sometimes not as palatable, some of this will also be addressed later in the book as practical experience.

The chances are a social worker from Adult Care will also make home visits to assess your needs, and that of the carer if it is a family member. This is also a starting point as far as equipment is concerned. In our case, we had on loan the hospital bed, mattress, a Manger Elk inflatable lifting cushion to assist in getting Cilla up off the floor following falls, a wheelchair, a narrow-gauged commode chair, a nebuliser and an adjustable bedside table. Towards the end of Cilla's life, it was necessary to suction out her mouth and upper throat, so a suctioning machine was also provided.

There are also, if you qualify, special needs grants, which can even include some building work if necessary. In our case, we were able to obtain a ceiling hoist, which is essential to some patients who have difficulty getting out of and back into bed. The hoist was professionally fitted and tested before being signed over for use. In our case, we were given an option to keep the hoist as ours and pay an annual maintenance fee, or sign the hoist over to the social provider in exchange for free annual maintenance. We chose the latter, since Cilla pointed out that once finished with, there was no need for us to keep it! I found the last half of the sentence in her quote telling and quite chilling...

Now here is the important, and probably the most crucial bit about having the equipment available at home and on-hand 24/7: *it allowed Cilla to stay at home!* I cannot stress this point too much, since I am convinced Cilla survived, overall, much longer than if she were in a nursing home.

Obviously, your doctor should already be in touch with you on a regular basis, and I also suggest you touch base with your local hospice. Even if you do not require their services as a resident, you will be amazed by what information and assistance they can offer. In Cilla's case, Dr Hume, and her predecessor Dr Jenks, from the Countess Mountbatten Hospice, were both available to discuss all manners of the illness. Also, and importantly, the chances are that any of the doctors at your local hospice will be familiar with PSP.

In our instance, before he transferred to Southampton's General Hospital, Dr Jenks made many home visits, drug consultations in conjunction with Cilla's doctor, and even donned a dress for Cilla.

To be fair, I need to quantify the latter part of that sentence...!

Cilla had a fantastic relationship with Dr Jenks, since they always appeared to be on the same wavelength. During one of their many informal discussions, it came about that Dr Jenks was going to be one of the leading 'ladies' in a future charity event being held locally. The event, held on the 9th of January 2015, was the pantomime, Robin Hood. In this instance, the carers took Cilla, and although Cilla could not see what was happening on stage, she loved the music and joined in the best she could when it came to arm waving. Once again, Georgie Huskins was on hand to take a series of photos and a series of short video clips.

Anyhow, to emphasis their relationship as doctor/patient, as soon as Dr Jenks found out that Cilla was in hospital for the final time, he did all he could to fulfil Cilla's last requests. He visited her bedside and got a welcoming smile and firm handhold from her, despite her circumstances.

I urge you to do all of this, and make first contact as soon as practicable. Remember, offer as much information as possible which, in turn, will help you establish a proper working relationship later.

And always remember the most important word in this section, which is: *communication!*

Nursing Homes

Now, I have already mentioned nursing homes, and I want to emphasis a point here that might, or might not, help you decide your own fate. Incidentally, I have chosen the term 'nursing home' as opposed to 'care home' because I found it more appropriate to Cilla's needs. This is not in any way designed to highlight either, but to make it easier for you to understand from our perspective.

Over the years, it was necessary for me to place Cilla in a nursing home so I could have a Respite break. I think it unfair to name any individual home because, within certain parameters, their main focus is on complying with the laws that govern their business. Ironically, out of all the words I used in the last sentence, to me, one stands out above all others: *business!*

It would be foolish to deny this point, since one of the first questions required to ask is: *What are the rates of stay?*

Do not get me wrong here, they provide an invaluable service to many; but I do question the relationship between the owners of the business and the people on the frontline. The dedicated people on the frontline are required to work for two masters: one being the business owners; the other, the residents. The real question is, as a frontline worker: *Who do you prioritise?*

It is true, certainly in our case, that not one of the nursing homes could provide a one to one care plan as achieved at home. Perhaps my parameters were far too high to start with, and when it is related to somebody you love and care about, then it becomes more personal – and by that I mean I know the person involved, their quirks, likes and needs. No matter how much time you devote to telling the frontline staff about these oddities, they will not have the same amount of time to devote their efforts to these idiosyncrasies.

It is logical that if it takes me and a home carer two hours to feed, shower, brush teeth and re-dress Cilla, then that is the benchmark for her care. However, for the nursing home staff to achieve this, do it properly, and in the same format as me, then with two staff to every six residents out of, say, thirty-six residents, it is going to take each frontline care pairing twelve man hours a day on this task alone. From this point of view, you can come to your own conclusions. Each nursing home has their own approach to caring, although the doctrines are basically the same; and to the business owners, each resident represents a pound for pound ratio and nothing more beyond that.

Perhaps I have been a little too harsh in my assessment, but here is the rub, and perhaps part of an alternative view. Nursing homes and care homes that specialise in dementia, often do not understand the characteristics of PSP, which unfortunately can easily be mistaken for an alternative illness. Given the peculiarities, if not properly informed, the staff who were not involved in the initial greeting procedures, might well assume that their 'charge' is suffering from dementia. In this instance, it might also be assumed that a PSP sufferer might be being awkward and not realistically understand the complexities surrounding them. I know that, in Cilla's case, she felt that she was being regarded in a way that would suggest such treatment. Indeed, she remembered many of the conversations that the 'staff' had in her presence, and which was highly inappropriate to somebody with full understanding.

For my part, and to help her in this instance, I placed a sign on the wall behind and above Cilla's head, which read:

HELLO – MY NAME IS CILLA

I DO NOT SUFFER FROM DEMENTIA BUT HAVE A VERY RARE ILLNESS CALLED *PSP*. THIS MEANS THAT I UNDERSTAND EVERYTHING BUT CANNOT COMMUNICATE WITH YOU THAT WELL.

EVERYTHING YOU SAY OR DO IN MY COMPANY IS UNDERSTOOD

Please do not get me wrong, in life I have worked under some extreme circumstances and, in some instances, deadlines were more important than human values, but this is also the case, in my mind, with the systems that control nursing home carers. They are all there because they want to 'make a difference', but in all honesty, their integrity is quite often taken for granted by the owners, which, in effect, dilutes or reduces their operational capabilities.

It is more than a matter of principle that I bring this example to your attention. I do it so you can, sooner rather than later, open up a dialogue about this extremely important factor.

Under the circumstances, Cilla's stay in the nursing homes was for no longer than two weeks. Unfortunately, on three of these occasions, the stay was enforced due to my own medical problems, and coincided with me being rushed into hospital with various ailments.

I suppose, the daily regime Cilla benefitted from at home was something I could never expect anybody else to live up to or by. To explain this further, I mean as time went by, I was convinced Cilla would eventually, and more rapidly, decline should she be subjected to any long-term stays away from home. In the Autumn of 2015, I was so concerned by this point that I reconsidered the whole approach to care. So much so that it was then that I considered having someone move into the house to look after her should I be away for any length of time. It is a decision I wished I had made much earlier!

Anyhow, as far as Cilla was concerned, her return home was always received with both relief *and* renewed respect for all of those carers who came to see her on a daily basis to tend to her needs.

Since dementia has been mentioned and is also relevant to PSP, I may as well put something to you that best describes my perception of the illness. Indeed, if I were asked to describe dementia to somebody who was reasonably well educated but ignorant of the fact that dementia existed, then the only and best way I could illustrate it, is to put it in this simplified analogy.

To clarify... for argument's sake, your main pleasure in life was to read your favourite book of all time. Furthermore, you were, through sheer pleasure, disposed to read it once a month and had done so for many years. However, over time and during each reading, ten words from the story were to randomly but temporarily disappear leaving no gaps... conversely, and occasionally another set of random words from the story would suddenly appear somewhere else in the book. Eventually, and over time, a combination of these words would disappear altogether and never come back to you at all. By the year's end, you as the reader would start to get confused by something once so familiar... so much so, that you would not know what to do.

Because it is your favourite book, however, you would remember most aspects of the story; but the sequence and, I believe, the main context of the book would eventually be lost to you. Ultimately though, the physical book itself would become blank and the story be wiped away altogether. In some cases, your favourite book would be replaced by another, less favourable to you.

Now, ask yourself this: As time goes on, and as these occurrences increased, what impact would that have on you?

My simplistic adaptation, is only meant to describe my version of the confusion one must suffer at the hands of this and other terrible neurological illnesses.

Day To Day

To highlight Cilla's needs, as mentioned under the last heading, I need to take you through a day in Cilla's life. Unless she was going out, then the schedule listed below was adhered to with absolute precision unless, of course, there were any unforeseen problems or unplanned trips... incidentally, forward planning is always essential!

One of the items of equipment loaned to us in conjunction with the bed was a Wendylett fitted base sheet. In fact, after a short period of time we increased that to two on loan, and at over £100 each they do not come cheap. The reason these were so important, was because Cilla had a penchant for nice things... and in her hour of need, who could blame her? One of her predilections was silk pyjamas, which, in conjunction with the aforementioned sheets, help us manoeuvre Cilla around the bed effortlessly.

I mention this because it is relevant to the overall image and now wish to portray her typical daily routine:

08:45 – Remove catheter night bag.

09:00 – Up out of bed – Breakfast. Meds. (*Due to its importance, I will cover the very significant topic of feeding later.*)

09:30 – Shower. Hair wash every third day unless requested otherwise.

10:30 – Back to bed, unless hair has been washed or the toilet is needed. However, in this instance, we aimed for 11:00 but fitted in with Cilla's needs accordingly.

Sleep.

13:30 – Up out of bed. Lunch. Meds. Cigarette.

15:00 – Back to bed, unless toilet is needed.

Sleep.

18:00 – Up out of bed. Tea. Meds. Cigarette.

19:30 – Back to bed, unless toilet is needed. Catheter night bag applied.

19:30-22:00 – Television.

22:00 – Meds. Settle down for the night.

I must point out that this was Cilla's daily schedule for most of the last two years of her life, and one that suited her. Prior to this, things were a little bit more flexible and reflected her essential needs and mobility at the time. As things progressed, it was necessary to add certain limitations, which in turn assisted Cilla in having a much more comfortable life.

In most cases, Cilla would be manually removed from her bed and elevated, with her full assistance, onto the commode chair. What made this operation so simple was Cilla's all-giving spirit to assist, and the lack of friction between Cilla and the aforementioned Wendylett fitted base sheet. With a small amount of effort and support, she just glided into position before swinging up into a sitting stance on the edge of the bed. Cilla would then slightly lean forward and raise her arms the best she could, before placing them on the shoulders of the carer. With the chair properly situated, it was then possible to raise her into a standing position.

This was always a moment for us to have what we called a 'huggle': *a combination of a hug and a cuddle.*

Once in the correct location, she would swing around before being lowered onto the seat. The reason a commode chair was used in these instances, was because it was the only mode of wheeled transport that would reach every room in the house due to its narrow width. You see, the required access into the kitchen was somewhat compromised by the distance between a built in oven and a kitchen worktop. This was due to the size of the kitchen, and the fact that these items were fixed and could not be accommodated anywhere else. Also, and although Cilla now saw dignity as something in her past life, she never used the commode as it was intended, just a way of getting around: a means to an end.

It is only fair that I now bring in the host of carers in Cilla's life; after all, they are a major part of the story. The carers were *all* individually mentioned at her funeral and are all cited in the front of this book – in both cases at Cilla's request.

But! Before I get to them, I must have a rant!

Should you decide to use a care company, what I write next is something you might, or might not, have already encountered yourselves. Importantly, what I write now is from the heart and based on personal experience. However, I would like to highlight this point once more: *This does not, and is not meant, to influence you! Whatever complements your needs are the most important factors in your own lives.*

In the beginning, we were allocated the services of a small private care firm, as at that time Cilla's needs were not as great as they eventually became. Due to the size of the company, the package and requirements from us, combined with Cilla's own capabilities at the time, worked extremely well. However, this was not always going to be the case due to business expansions, buy-outs, and where Cilla's ever-changing needs were concerned.

In the latter stages of Cilla's care, we often found conflict with the management within the companies who, much like the nursing homes, had different objectives and constraints to that of the girls 'out in the field'. In fact, Cilla and I 'discussed' this at length one day and, in our opinion, the system was flawed. We both agreed that in some cases, the management were more inclined to work for the company than the client, which within itself is a perilous permutation.

For example, the distance between the neighbouring village of Hedge End and our home address in West End, is 1.8 miles and on a perfect day within a seven-minute time-frame. Unfortunately, between Hedge End and West End is a major road artery: The M27. Although the girls coming from Hedge End – usually their last call before ours – did not use the M27, they still had to cross two major feeder roads. At peak times, and due to the usual heavy traffic, accidents and incidents, the roads often backed up beyond these boundaries. To make matters worse, during the cricket season and concert or event evenings at the Ageas Bowl, which is located between the two villages, the traffic increased twenty-fold. To add to the problem, often between certain times during the applicable evenings, the roads were closed. This meant a lengthy detour for the girls, which added two miles and up to thirty minutes to their journey and already tight schedule.

The reason for the geography lesson is to show what the girls had to deal with, since the management involved generally only allowed one to five minutes between each scheduled call. But each call, in the worst-case scenario, could subsequently lose up to twenty minutes of care due to this – much to the dismay of both carers and 'client', as we were usually referred as. This discrepancy in time is commonly known in the care business as 'clipping'! The name derives from the necessity of the girls to clip up to ten minutes off their current call to try and get to their next client on time. In reality, it works both ends of the spectrum, since they often left their previous call ten minutes early due to the pressures they were under, and would arrive ten minutes late to us at the other end.

Due to this, and other pressures, there is often a huge turnover of staff, which means either cancellations or, at worst, the involvement of agency staff. Given the right set of circumstances, and in a perfect environment, there is absolutely nothing wrong with agency staff; however, how they are used by the care companies is often detrimental to us, the clients.

In our case, agency staff sometimes turned up without notice and were expected to deal with Cilla and her complex needs without adequate information. Unfortunately, in these instances, it was necessary for me to show them the intricacies involved, whilst with little input from them they stood and watched. The vast majority of the time this would be the last time we would see that particular duo. Likewise, the next day, another unknown pairing would turn up and I would have to repeat the whole process again. To compound the issue, the agency staff were, more often than not, on double the hourly rate our regular girls were on.

One particular request that Cilla had put forward in all of the care packages was that she did not want men carers. Of course, I complied with this request as I would any other... ! However, where the agency workers were concerned, they received no such instruction from the care company, and on several occasions a man would turn up, only to be told to wait well away from the personal care side of things.

There was also the issue of security and safety. In one instance, an agency worker had been given access to the outside key safe code, and just entered the house unannounced. I do not know what security checks are in place by the care company, but their regular staff always had the courtesy to knock first, since it was generally known that I was always ready to answer the door. As a result, I became more aware of this problem and started to change the key safe codes more frequently.

Incidentally, these points have all been well considered before being added to the contents of this book, since it would have been remiss of me not to include any pitfalls involved.

Now for the positive aspects!

What you are about to read in this following section mainly involves dedication and selective nepotism on my part. Some people impacted on Cilla's life so much, that I cannot go on without mentioning them individually.

In principle, the overall relationship with the regular carers could not have been any better. In the vast majority of the cases, these relationships grew solely on the basis of Cilla's good nature, natural ability to put people at ease, and her wicked sense of humour. These instinctive characteristics built within Cilla's own psyche instantly put them, the carers, and anybody else for that matter, at ease from the start.

In the beginning, Cilla was allocated a ten-and-a-half-hour a week care package, and it is worth mentioning that my own health is generally poor, and without their assistance, I would have struggled... in fact, I did!

Despite this, I promised Cilla that she would never live her final days in a nursing home, and am extremely proud to have been able to keep that promise.

Bid and Pauline were two of the first carers to have had contact with Cilla, and as with all the carers past and future, they bonded straight away. It does my heart good to think back to those days, hearing a variety of songs being sung with gusto coming from the bathroom and well above the sound of the shower. Mostly, due to the age of Bid and Pauline, the songs were something Cilla could relate to, since this was also another one of Cilla's passions. Cilla knew many of the songs word for word, line by line, and could at that stage, and within reason, join in.

Once Bid and Pauline had left the scene for pastures new, we were allocated much younger carers. At first, I was sceptical about their abilities, so became pensive when it came to personal care. I need not have worried, since I am convinced Cilla's general demeanour played its part in putting the new girls at ease. Once again, I could hear both singing and excessive laughter coming from within the confines of the bathroom. This general attitude from the girls easily matched Cilla's sense of fun.

All in all, I can honestly say that the majority of the girls who came to care for Cilla on a day-to-day basis did exactly that: they cared for her! It was like they were all buddies, and soon formed friendships rather than a client-carer role. This correlation is proved by the list of honour in the front of the book, and as I have already said, Cilla wanted them to know how strongly she felt about their role in her day-to-day care; indeed, her life!

Also, it appeared that the girls adapted to the situation around themselves and subsequently developed their own routines, which included various forms of therapy.

To give you an example, in the latter years, a few of the girls discovered a slight quirk in Cilla's progressive development. The quirk in question, was her lack of ability to throw! This was an accidental discovery, and one that amused Cilla as much as anybody else.

To see if they could help, the girls rolled up a few sheets of kitchen towel into a ball and asked Cilla to throw it to them. It appeared that this was impossible to her, since no matter how she held it, she could not let it go! Then they asked if she could drop it onto the floor or into their hand... the outcome was the same. Remarkably, both sides saw this as a challenge, and I could see in Cilla's eyes, both sheer determination and a sense of fun. She never was able to throw the tissue, but never ever gave up trying!

In all though, caring as far as the girls were concerned, was much more than frivolity, as they were acutely serious in the overall care.

On more than one occasion, arrangements were made between themselves to do things mostly shunned by management, and in some instances, certain professional bodies. For instance, as a cigarette smoker Cilla took great pleasure in smoking, and it was occasionally the girl's responsibility to oversee this. After a short while, some of the girls were fervently encouraged by Cilla to join in, and to be fair, some did not need too much encouragement. Enclosed within the confines of the kitchen, and with the back door wide open, I could once again hear nothing but laughter and merriment coming from within.

From this, small talk developed, and in no time at all they would be discussing anything and everything related to whatsoever. Primarily, I was not involved in these periods of high spirits, but Cilla loved the camaraderie, and it also seemed that no subject was taboo either! This was soon to become known as 'girlie talk', to which I was further excluded, and provided Cilla with a sense of belonging which, I am sure, took her back to her days at work.

In no time at all, nothing became too much trouble for them, and the girls instantly offered to spend their free time making Cilla's life that little bit more comfortable.

What made this observation more poignant was that the less professional they became, the more Cilla liked the situation, because she now felt that she was among friends. Interestingly, although some of the professional constraints had been put to one side, her care improved and, as far as the girls were concerned, nothing seemed like too much trouble.

Believe me, these were not isolated incidents, since Cilla had an aptitude of inspiring pretty much every carer into doing the same, and subtly seducing them into her world. By now, I guess you have noticed that I cannot stress enough the power of Cilla's persona. I also cannot stress enough the power of Cilla's individuality and her natural likeability, even when she was at her most vulnerable.

To be fair, personal care is something that, under normal circumstances, stays personal, and usually does not involve anybody else. But unfortunately, when somebody is in Cilla's position, personal care becomes a necessity. Cilla once said something quite telling about her understanding of the situation: *'Dignity comes second place to cleanliness.'*

This observation on her part is almost certainly true, which I am certain is why the correlation between carer and client cannot always remain impassive. Truly, if you are inclined by nature to take up care as a profession, then by the very same nature that enticed you into the profession, you will ultimately feel affection for the person you are caring for... especially if you are as meritorious as Cilla was.

I specifically mentioned a few of the girls under the headings 'Carers – Special Mention' and 'Carers – Beyond the Call of Duty'. Whilst this sounds elitist, it is not meant to be, since I would have loved to have given examples of each and every one of them: like Kate Haines singing David Essex songs, and her crazy stories about her antics at Stompers; or Abby and Dale-Anne talking enthusiastically about their respective horses, which Cilla enjoyed hearing about since her own experiences came to the fore.

However, this is not possible... perhaps in another book! So I shall continue with the intention of showing how some of these girls actually cared.

In the first category, I have mentioned the following: Stacey Humphrey, Bobbie Ribeiro, Rose Jones and Naomi Gibbs.

If I were able to show you a hundred photographs of Cilla, you would notice many things about her, but none more so than the various hairstyles she sported over the years. Despite Cilla's illness, she expected no less of herself than the best when it came to cleanliness and appearance. This was plain to see, and the girls knew it, especially when they knew Cilla was due to go out for whatever the reason. In these instances, Stacey would come to the house in her own time, and being an ex-hairdresser, would prepare Cilla's hair for the day. Plaits, bunches, experimental designs were all available, and nothing seemed too much of a problem. Even temporary colour was applied for one occasion, and an outside source once affixed a feather interweave which Stacey regularly maintained, much to the gratitude of Cilla.

Bobbie was Cilla's most regular Take a Break sitter, and would frequently forward plan their days ahead – although sitter, in this instance, is a bit of a misleading term because sitting was something they did less frequently than not! In many cases, Bobbie would take Cilla out in her wheelchair to the local garden centre, Haskins. Here, they would plot and plan between themselves all manner of things to do in the garden. Also, due to Cilla's illness, many people were stumped when it came to giving her birthday and Christmas presents, so, Haskins vouchers were always suggested on her behalf, and eventually became the norm. With these, it was possible for her to purchase whatever she wanted within their extensive range, which mostly included items designated for her precious garden. Between them, and whilst out, they would also have tea and cake, which in Cilla's case included her favourite: a rum baba!

These days out were so precious to Cilla and always remembered with the fondest of memories. Bobbie oversaw these most pleasurable days for over two years before, sadly, having to stop due to injuries sustained in a car accident whilst on holiday in America.

Now I have mentioned Cilla's garden and her Haskins purchases, I shall now introduce you to both Rose and Naomi. Once more, these girls took it upon themselves to give up their precious free time to plant out some of Cilla's many purchases. In this instance, 360 plant bulbs were embedded in various pots. Not only did they plant them out, they regularly nurtured them with water, love and tender care. Cilla was most impressed with their efforts and, for one season and given her fading eyesight, she was able to see and smell their startling results. They even went one stage further by organising a day out to Beaulieu, where Cilla would make her final visit to the place she still loved and cared for; and when I say they, I include Naomi, Rose and Georgie, along with Cilla. Oh, how I would have loved to have eavesdropped on that eventful day.

With perfect weather, in Rose's cabriolet car and the roof down, they had a wonderful time, where I understand, Cilla was able to point out various places of interest and reminisced the best she could. It was a wonderful sensation to see the glow on Cilla's cheeks and the sparkle in her eyes when they finally returned.

Going on from here, Cilla has a lot of people to thank in her overall care, but none more so than three carers in particular. I have classed these as 'Carers – Beyond the Call of Duty', and for very good reason!

Georgie Huskins, Hannah Foster and Kerrie Potter are amongst the noblest of people I know:

straight to the point, and without personal agendas.

Following a change in direction with Cilla's care, Hannah and Kerrie assisted Georgie in her now full-time capacity as carer. Georgie had always been involved with Cilla's care, but eventually took over the day-to-day care due to failings within the care company last involved in Cilla's daily and personal upkeep. In each case, I would leave them to get on with things, and in the background I would hear chatter, laughter and music.

Incidentally, to prove her worth, Hannah actually resigned from her previous employers, just so she could remain as Cilla's carer.

Between Georgie, Hannah and Kerrie, Cilla could not have been in better hands.

And talking of hands, apart from Cilla's hair, she had another defining feature: her nails! Without fail, and even if I was away for a short break or abroad, Georgie would make arrangements for Cilla to have her nails renewed with acrylic and painted in the brightest, glitteriest coloured nail polish on the shelves. These were her showpiece, and towards the end of her life, she added one significant attribute mainly due to some weight loss: as her fingers slimmed down, she was unable to wear her wedding ring and chose to have her ring finger nail painted gold, no matter what the colour or design on the other fingers. Likewise, with the exception of her wedding finger, and over Christmas, she would always have alternate green glittered and red glittered nails. This was her homage to the Christmas spirit, and a way of saying, *'I'm here, and I am still beautiful!'* Because she could not drive, Georgie was not alone in this enterprise since she often recruited the help of Naomi Gibbs in my absence.

In Kerrie's case, she would keep Cilla informed of day to day activities and more often than not, keep Cilla informed about her own family. Cilla was always keen to hear what goes on in each of the carers households, since she then felt part of a much larger group... almost like an unofficial family member.

Despite everything I have emphasised, this is not to say that any of the other carers would not have done anything different than all I have highlighted before; in fact, given the opportunity, I know they would.

I think you have, by now, got the purpose of my sentiments, so I shall keep this final piece about carers brief.

These tributes might seem strange in a book of this type, but I am only doing as promised by highlighting the issues I discussed with Cilla during the last years of her life... and for that, I am eternally grateful to have had this opportunity. In fact, it was something she felt needed to be accentuated because, fortunately, most of us have options when it comes to care. In each case, the little social gifts the girls gave Cilla are exactly what makes these individual carers exceptional.

Between Cilla and I, we came to the conclusion that, if practicable, care in your own environment is by far better than any nursing home: *there is definitely no place like home!*

I think it only fair to point out that by the time Cilla passed, she was allocated forty-three-and-a-half hours a week of home care, plus full support from all of the associated agencies involved.

Once more, before I move on, you might recall my little rant earlier. As with all things in life, we all have theories, and I am no exception. So in line with my views, I have two words in response to both nursing homes and care agencies: *John Lewis!*

In my humble opinion, the main reasons they – nursing homes and care agencies – continually fail, is because of the way the management is structured: trying to separate who actually works for who is almost impossible. Under normal circumstances, businesses around the world work well within a filter down management structure, but it appears to have the opposite effect in the world of care.

You see, John Lewis has a policy structure that involves partnerships from the top to the bottom, and the strategy actually works. If it did not, then how and why does John Lewis succeed to the highest levels?

If only care organisations were to adopt this working philosophy, then perhaps there would be an improvement. Instead of profits being channelled one way, once costs have been taken into account, they could simply be evenly divided.

The bottom line is that everybody would be working as a collective, with the clients being the sole subject of their success. Can you imagine anyone within the group not wanting to do well for their client if it meant that they too would suffer as a result?

The second biggest winner, after the client, would be the down-to-earth, day-to-day, run of the mill carer.

If everybody, including top management, were to work together and for the same end, then the care profession would succeed. I am afraid to say that I have only seen it from one perspective and, sadly, that is where a faceless organisation puts profits first.

However, to sum up everything I have said about 'hands on' carers and Cilla's impact upon them, I include these final principles. This time though, these values are in the words of some of the carers I have already mentioned:

Kate Haines recently recalled her feelings and the impression Cilla made upon her:

'In all my years of working in social care, Cilla was one of the bravest, strongest and most courageous women I have ever met. No matter how she was feeling, she had the best sense of humour ever and always had the biggest smile... I just wish I got to know her for longer.'

Hannah Foster expressed how she felt following the loss of Cilla:

'*I feel so privileged to have known such a wonderful woman, both inside and out. Thinking of her as often as I do, always brings a smile to my face.*'

Georgie Huskins – rarely lost for words – added this:

'*To say Cilla had an impact on my life would be an understatement. It feels like I have known her all my life... I miss her each and every day. All I have left are photographs and happy memories.*'

Stacey Humphrey gave me this personal analysis since Cilla made such an impact on her:

'*I have suffered greatly with losses in my life, but none more so than somebody who crept into my life through work. Cilla was different in so many ways... she gave dignity and courage a new meaning. She loved me doing her hair and I felt privileged to be able to make this small contribution for this beautiful woman.*'

Caring Families

I have already mentioned professional carers and the role they play, but what about us... the family?

Questions: Could you care for a loved one who is terminal? What does it take to become a carer? Are family members trained to care? Or are we all natural-born carers? I ask this, even if your own circumstances are not best placed due to other commitments.

Now, the questions above are not meant to provoke a response, but merely to ask if you, as an individual, have it in you to care for a loved one with the knowledge they are going to die? Not only are they going to die, but will die within a certain amount of time and in increments over a matter of years? Certainly, at what point does the issue even exist?

Actually, asking if you have it in you to care for somebody who is dying is impossible to answer! In fact, how can anyone possibly answer a series of questions like that without actually being put into a position that requires it to happen first? Outside care has to be taken into account, as well as other important personal details, such as providing for your own family. Importantly, you must not feel bad if you are unable to provide such care, no matter what I have already said. Each and every case must be analysed accordingly, and on merit... your own individual circumstances will partly make that decision for you.

Some illnesses provoke violent responses in the most amiable of people. How do you account for that? Others require acute medical care, which within itself is almost impossible to achieve outside hospitals and hospices. The fact is, I do not envy anybody finding themselves in these positions.

And, as I have already explained, Cilla made my task easy!

In today's society, we would all like to think that we would care for a loved one, and with absolute conviction in their time of need. Under normal circumstances, and if pressed for a response, then the majority of people would acknowledge the original question with ease and a resounding yes... But until the time comes, you do not actually know, and one only has to read the news to see that this is often the case.

Take me as an example.

Never in a million years could I ever have imagined myself in the role of carer. Up until Cilla's illness, and only when the issue was raised by other people, would I ponder the question of caring. In real terms and in my day-to-day life as it was, I would have considered it well outside my scope. In fact, at one time, the interpretation of the word carer only ever extended to caring *about* somebody, not actually caring *for* somebody. To me it meant to love the person you are with, and to treat them with respect and within a certain set of parameters. These parameters, or feelings, sat in line with the person I was with at the time. If I am honest with myself, I would have to admit that I was more selfish with my feelings than I would have liked to have been: I actually believed that the stronger the physical relationship, the stronger the care I felt for the person.

Surprisingly, despite Cilla's previous illnesses and restrictions, I did not see myself as being in a caring role until PSP entered our lives. Indeed, even when I did eventually take over as Cilla's eyes, mouth, legs and other related areas that no longer worked, I did not consciously think about it. I suppose, with PSP being progressive, it makes it slightly more acceptable to become a carer, since one minute you are speaking to each other and the next you have adapted a whole new language using signs.

One could express opinions all day about the subject, but to be fair it was PSP that actually helped me realise my potential. As strange as that statement seems, my theory is purely based on the fact that the illness is progressive. Unlike a stroke or any other sudden medical issue, PSP allows the carer, in this case me, time to slowly develop an understanding of both the person I cared for and the illness. As one issue arose I dealt with it, and then bit by bit, as it increased in its severity, I found the next stage easier to understand and adapted accordingly.

I suppose, when you look back on Cilla's previous medical history, you realise that this too happened in increments and was easily lost in time.

Of course, as I have already mentioned, there was something else in my favour: *Cilla!*

Cilla never made a fuss, and actually put a lot of effort in helping me help her. PSP has a tendency to provoke either anger or apathy in the patient, and in Cilla's case, it was apathy. Ironically, this was in line with her genetic coding and natural philosophy, since she was always so laid back about life itself. She was never one to panic or make a fuss about any given situation, and could often be accused of being far too relaxed about some things. Cilla certainly had a calming influence, and much like her ability to start a party with her arrival, she could also calm a situation in a similar way.

If I might be so bold... if it were at all possible, I strongly suggest that you base your care for others on the one person you know best: *yourself!*

Ask yourself one question: *How would I like to be treated?*

There can only be one answer to that question, which brings me to the same conclusion: *care for others as you would care for yourself.*

I will give you an example of what I mean.

It did not occur to me straight away, but one morning while feeding Cilla, I had an itchy nose. With a spoon in one hand and a bowl in the other, I persevered until the sensation finally went. Occasionally, during this time, I would wrinkle my nose as a form of relief, and then it hit me: *How does Cilla clear her nose or scratch an itch?*

I regularly blow mine into a tissue, but Cilla did not have that capacity. After breakfast, and following a short discussion, I cleared Cilla's nostrils. I did this by use of a corner section of a baby wipe, rolled to a fine but blunt point, and applied some gentle prodding and teasing. As gross as this might sound to some, there was both a look of contentment on Cilla's face, and relief once finished. This, thereafter, became part of our daily routine, and one she thoroughly appreciated.

Before Cilla became ill, she bathed daily, dressed smartly, wore fresh clean underwear each and every day, brushed her teeth at least twice a day, and always looked after her hair and nails. So why should that change just because she could not do it for herself? As a result of this knowledge – and let us face facts, if you know your loved one then you would already know these details – I was able to formulate a plan around her own personal hygiene.

I have mentioned Cilla's silk pyjamas already, but what I did not say is that she had them changed daily. Likewise, her knickers and socks too. Since I have mentioned socks, I should explain that for many years prior to the illness getting hold, Cilla suffered from cold feet. This may well have something to do with poor circulation and her many back operations, although I am not entirely sure of this point. However, I made sure there was an ample supply of everything she could possibly need, including socks!

Essentially there was one large cupboard in her room that contained a vast supply of all her toiletries, tissues and scents. This was dubbed by the girls, as 'the shop', and they all knew that if they removed anything from the shop, then it was to go onto the shopping list. As a result of this obligatory system, Cilla never ran out of any one product, ever!

Before I commence, I wish to remind you of one of Cilla's quotes: *'Dignity comes second place to cleanliness.'*

Accompanying this thought, there is another need I have not previously referred to – and believe me, I pondered deeply on this subject before deciding to mention it – is toilet matters!

You can take these two words in any way you want, but yes... toilet matters... and a great deal in fact! And toilet matters as a means to describe a function. In both cases, they are relevant and pertinent to this next point.

Cilla, as you know, was fitted with a catheter, so the subject here is purely related to bowel movements. As a rule, Cilla required my assistance, above all others, when she needed to have a poo. She would be placed onto the toilet, never the commode, and left with a gardening kneeling pad under her feet for warmth, and a largish pillow between the left-hand side of her head and the bathroom wall.

It was essential for Cilla to use the pillow to rest her head upon, since the space between the toilet and the wall is only ten inches.

When she required further assistance, she tapped the closest handrail or radiator with the cleaning brush which was always within her reach. On entering the bathroom, she would show me either one finger or two. One would signify a single set of gloves and two would signify two sets of gloves depending on the consistency of her bowel movement. Due to the lack of day-to-day movement and exercise, it was very difficult to balance her bowel medication. This meant that there were times when she needed light and sensitive assistance, hence two sets of gloves. Also, since she was unable to wipe herself clean, this was also taken into account.

I will not dwell on this point, but Cilla would deliberately hold back if I was unavailable, and only ask one other in extreme cases: Georgie, at a push (no pun intended), would be asked on the rarest of occasions to assist in this matter. The intimacy involved in this process can only be shared by somebody who you truly trust and someone who truly cares... ask any mother!

If there was any reason at all to mention what I have written above, it is to highlight the dedication one must have in these situations, and to emphasise how far you must be prepared to go in looking after someone.

Likewise, it also shows Cilla's dedication in getting her story across and to open boundaries which some are sometimes too afraid to speak of. Once again, she knew this subject was going to be confronted, and also knew that only good could possibly come from sharing.

She wanted you to know that to be a sufferer or a carer, then all aspects of this and other illnesses must be understood and spoken about freely, which brings me onto the next point: *feeding!*

Feeding

B efore I continue and give you details about Cilla's eating habits and how PSP changed her regime, I have to mention her abilities as a cook.

The very first meal she presented to me on a plate was chips, tomato, beetroot and blue cheese. Now there is no way I will ever forget that combination, especially as it was presented to me at two in the morning... but I must say, it was not only memorable, but absolutely delicious.

From here, she explored and diversified before becoming a bit more traditional. Our first Sunday roast was a huge success; although I was not party to the development or knowledgeable about the background of its success until months later. Apparently, this was the first time Cilla had become so adventurous with food, and after preparing everything, she phoned her mother for help. Bit by bit, telephone call after telephone call, the plot and the gravy thickened, and by the time it was presented, Cilla was exhausted... and I did notice the pensive looks coming my way as I took the first mouthful of her roast beef. Delicious!

It appeared she was a natural, and from there on, she devised her own recipes. Incredibly, if a roast dinner could get any better, then I would not have believed it if I had not tasted it for myself. Yes, as a cook, she was an unmitigated success!

Strangely, I can remember that first meal she ever prepared for me, but sadly, and although nearer in time, I cannot remember the last.

Generally, Cilla was a meat eater – although that all changed one hot day in 1987 due to a casual, if not enforced, observation. Following a lengthy trip, and due to an accident further up the road from us on the M5, we and the associated traffic were crawling along at under ten miles an hour. Now that should not have had anything to do with meat within itself; however, alongside us for many miles was a lorry transporting live chickens, and we could not escape the combination of smell, noise and feathers filling the air. With Cilla seated closest to the enclosed mayhem, and with the car windows wide open due to the heat, she made a firm resolution: *no more meat!*

For some unknown reason, she excluded seafood from this statement and chose to eat vegetarian and seafood only. From that day forth she became a devout pescetarian.

I have to admit, I feared for my future Sunday roasts and Wednesday chops, but I need not have worried as despite her newfound outlook on food, Cilla continued to handle, cook and serve meat to me, and any of our many guests who knew about her ability to cook.

True to her word, Cilla stuck to her programme; which was not too surprising, as once she had made her mind up over a subject, she invariably stuck to it... possibly with the exception of smoking.

Anyhow, in the earliest stages of PSP, Cilla developed a taste for three cheese and red onion sandwiches. At first, Cilla would eat the same filled sandwiches for lunch without assistance, or change the menu for months on end. Later it would become prawn sandwiches. Anyways, the crust would be nibbled around, and the dogs would gratefully eat whatever was left over. In time, Cilla found it difficult to hold the sandwiches and asked me to cut the edges off – which was no problem. Eventually, I ended up cutting the sandwiches into small cubes, which Cilla appreciated, and found the bite-sized portions fairly easy to chew. Then, after about two years, Cilla found chewing and swallowing – bread in particular – more difficult, and decided to change her culinary delights from sandwiches to omelettes. Omelettes seemed to suit her palate and she experimented with various soft fillings, such as mushrooms. Once more, it was necessary to cut the food up into bite-sized portions.

It was now that I noticed Cilla was having difficulty raising her arm up high enough to reach her mouth. As with the case with a child, I found she required assistance and started to feed her. Her chewing technique had slowed too, and swallowing became more difficult as the months went by. It got to the point where she could no longer sustain a proper chewing action, so I looked for alternative foods.

From here we were much restricted by what was available off-the-shelf, since I was also limited by what I could physically cook. Of course, some would say cook a large amount of whatever and freeze for future use. Don't get me wrong, I am... sorry, was... a brilliant cook as Cilla helped me develop my cooking skills early in the marriage. It was just that I was limited by physical constraints, and apart from having restricted physical abilities, I was also too busy organising Cilla's day, despite the help I was getting. Of course, the girls were willing to step in, and indeed the majority of the omelettes were cooked by them, but I also needed them to concentrate on Cilla's other needs. Gratefully, Rose Jones, also a dedicated pescetarian, even went one stage further and prepared the occasional meal for Cilla from her own home.

The end result was, of course, baby food heated in the microwave. Self-contained and ready to heat, they were the ideal alternative to her normal foods. I was, however, surprised by two things when buying baby food: first, the price seemed a little excessive for the portion sizes, and secondly, there were more meat-based meals than vegetarian. It appears baby produce and baby products, along with anything to do with the disabled, is charged at a premium... Just another personal view.

Incidentally, on closer inspection, we found that even baby food needed to be blended due to the amount of bits of hard vegetables involved, and these bits were something Cilla could certainly not cope with.

By the way, I must mention another important point that is relevant to feeding, but involves fluids.

Cilla detested thickeners and refused all drinks that contained it. This made me think about alternatives, and the only one drink I could entice her with was one I have already mentioned: mango juice.

Mango juice has a mix of positive attributes, but none more so than its natural thickness. Here was a juice that I could add her crushed and powdered medication to without loss of their essential powers, as the crushed powder would sit on top of the juice and slowly be absorbed before a final stir. There was never any residue left in the glass afterwards, and if wholly swallowed, then you have full knowledge that the dose given had been completely taken.

Breakfasts consisted mainly of fluids and were made up of a mix of juices and flavoured breakfast shakes. Incidentally, in the early stages, Cilla's favourite breakfast was porridge sweetened with honey. Anyhow, when feeding Cilla these drinks, it was necessary to have a steady hand – and even steadier nerve. It was necessary to balance and tilt, whilst monitoring the intake all at the same time. Too much tilt would often result in choking and spillage, so I found standing slightly behind Cilla, with our shoulders almost together the most effective position. Part of the problem was that Cilla became a guzzler and, as a collective, the carers and I had to slow her down. On occasions, Cilla would slightly raise her hand to the bottom of the tumbler and push upwards. When this happened, I felt worried about her breathing, and had to physically slow the process down when she became so demanding. In these instances, she would end up almost out of breath – similar to someone who had just completed an intensive run!

Straws were never a viable option, since her ability to suck had long since gone. Indeed, in the early days when I tried Cilla with a straw, the sucking reflex was there, but the fluid hit the back of her throat far too quickly for her body to react: in other words, her powers to swallow were being compromised because her sluggish reactions had slowed down the physical process, and fluids arrived at a juncture well before her body could respond.

Nonetheless, the importance of these daily fluid intakes was evident in her healthy skin tone and elasticity. Often I would lightly pinch the skin on the back of her hand to see how it reacted. This simple test was eventually carried out daily, and if the skin returned to its original position straight away, then I knew everything was okay. However, during this test, if the skin remained peaked for some time afterwards, then the signs are telling you that dehydration is, or could be, the case. Either way, I strongly suggest this test is implemented into your daily routine.

I also supplemented her prescribed medication with two other forms of treatment. Firstly, due to her lack of mobility, I gave her a daily dose of a single Aspirin, and secondly, a cranberry tablet. The Aspirin helped keep her blood thinned, and the cranberry assisted in the avoidance of UTIs.

Cilla also had a daily dose of cranberry juice, which she tolerated at a pinch as in each case she recognised the benefits.

Incidentally, since some people had suggested to me that it might be possible to use an oral 'feeding' syringe direct into the mouth, I would like to stress caution. Much like my reference to drinking straws... it is still possible to promotion choking even if pureed food is directed to the side wall of the mouth.

Anyhow, it was now, and due to her lack of control over swallowing, that we had to discuss more important issues since they appeared to be fast approaching.

Question: *What happens when you can no longer swallow properly?*

However, before you answer the question and before you as a reader, family member or sufferer 'peg it' – you will soon get the inference – contemplate carefully, and take the following details into deep consideration... certainly try to fully understand the entirety of the consequences first.

Please forgive the flippant remark in the earlier sentence, but I needed your undivided attention for what you are about to read... and I am sure I now have it.

There is a very strong reason for leaving this delicate subject to the latter end of the book, because if you remember nothing else, you must remember this next section. Encapsulated within its content, is a powerful reminder of who we are and what we are capable of. Why? Because initially, to think that we are always doing the right thing needs a lot more consideration than what our heart tells us. Next, you need do no more than read a story strongly linked to Cilla, and how she coped with a certain situation to fully understand my meaning.

Therefore, I respectfully dedicate this next section to Colin Browes and his family.

Peg Feeding

C oincidentally, or should I say crucially, a link appeared on the internet and later highlighted on one of the PSP pages relating to this very subject. I had to read it twice before deciding to read it to Cilla, as it had all sorts of connotations and considerations to take into account.

The following is just as much a dedication and tribute to a fellow sufferer of PSP as it is for all other sufferers. Without him, or his family's devotion towards him as a parent and as an adored father, then I am convinced that Cilla would not have taken the decision she finally did.

I have, with absolute gratitude, gained permission from Niki Browes and her family, as well as the editorial team at the publishers of *Daily Mail OnLine*, to reproduce the following article in its entirety. The heading is theirs, and the story is straight from the heart, and is replicated exactly as per the article:

I COULDN'T LOVE DAD MORE – BUT NOW I WISH I'D LET HIM DIE

Published: Daily Mail OnLine 00:10, 10 May 2012

By Niki Browes

'When her adored father was struck down by a brain disease, Niki agreed to him being kept alive by a feeding tube. So why does she now think it's the cruellest thing she's ever done?

One of my favourite memories of my father is of him tall and strikingly handsome in a grey morning suit, his arm linked into mine, on my sister's wedding day. He looks strong, vigorous and is beaming with fatherly pride.

Now, as I write this, Dad sits in a care home in Yorkshire, his eyes clamped shut, his chin slumped on to his chest, unable to eat, drink or move. He cannot talk.

All that remains is his hearing and a tenuous sense of who I am. He is 63 – yet he's a mere shell of the sporty, gregarious man he used to be. All I want for my dad Colin now is for death to release him from the prison of his suffering. But his life – against my will – is being artificially prolonged.

For a year, since Dad lost the capacity to chew and swallow, he has been kept alive by a tube that feeds him – known as a PEG tube – and the law prevents us from removing it.

So Dad is not permitted to slip seamlessly from this half-life into perpetual sleep.

Instead, a crueller death awaits him: he will be sustained by nutrients pumped into him until he chokes on his own saliva or dies of pneumonia.

Dad has a rare, untreatable brain disease called Progressive Supranuclear Palsy (PSP). For the past six years it has progressively stripped him of his humanity.

First he lost his strength and co-ordination; then his mental acuity deserted him.

He became doubly incontinent, he has difficulty opening his eyes, and the last words he said to me – 14 months ago – were a whispered: 'I love you'.

As the capacity to eat and drink began to desert him, my brother Ben, 25, and I – his next-of-kin – were encouraged by the management of his care home to have a PEG fitted.

My instinct was to resist – years earlier Dad had said to me: 'If ever I'm ill, please push me over a cliff' – but he was wasting away.

At 6ft 1in tall, he weighed just 10 stone – and it was awful to see him so visibly diminished and frail.

So although his level of understanding was questionable and he could not speak, I asked him if he wanted to be fed through a tube.

His response was to raise his thumb. So Ben and I agreed: the PEG should be fitted.

When we made the decision, we did not know it would be irrevocable. We were not told the law would prevent us from reversing it, even if Dad's pain became untenable.

It is a profound regret that I did not research the legal implications of our decision.

Our father now is such a pale shadow of the man he once was; it is utterly heart-breaking. He and my mum, Anne, were a glamorous, affluent, outgoing couple, and although they divorced when I was 21, Mum still visits him.

Dad was 24 when I was born, and was a wonderful, devoted father.

It was he who came to my bedside to soothe me when I had nightmares as a child. I remember him stroking my hair and staying with me until I fell asleep again.

He was a successful businessman and was managing director of a succession of prosperous businesses. Our home, in a pretty Derbyshire village, was a converted stable block.

Dad was always well-groomed and immaculately dressed and loved to zip around country lanes in his Jaguar. Sport was his passion and his favourite afternoons were whiled away at the village cricket club.

Fitness was almost an obsession: he played his beloved cricket, and squash, until his mid-50s when the first signs of his illness appeared.

It is now eight years since I noticed the first, insidious signs of the disease. I was then an editor on a men's magazine and had a two-seater sports car to review.

As Dad had always owned powerful cars I drove up to see him; I knew he'd love to take a spin.

But it was a shock to see him struggle in and out of the car. He must have noticed my concern because he laughed, blaming his stiffness on a vigorous game of squash.

The disease continued on its remorseless course. In New Year 2004, when Dad and I went to New Zealand to visit my sister Rachel and her children, its effects were too obvious to ignore. He would ask me to do up the buttons on his polo shirt; he could no longer tie his own shoelaces.

Back in England, I urged him to visit his GP. He was diagnosed, at first, with Parkinson's disease – he was just 55 – but when his condition deteriorated rapidly, a second opinion revealed that he had PSP.

His sharp physical decline was accompanied by a loss of co-ordination; his perception became dulled, his faculties less acute.

Having recently split up with his long-term partner – Ben's mum – Dad had bought a cottage in a remote village outside Doncaster.

A proud man to the last, he resisted our pleas to stop driving.

But when he wrote off his new 4x4 – thankfully harming no one but himself – to our huge relief he surrendered his driving licence.

And the drugs he was taking for his symptoms had an unwelcome side-effect.

He became uncharacteristically reckless with his finances. Dad, a successful businessman, was suddenly vulnerable; easy prey to the unscrupulous.

In the end, his cottage was repossessed. By then on state benefits, Dad spent some time in sheltered accommodation for those with progressive illnesses.

But, free to come and go as he pleased, and increasingly delusional, he often put himself in harm's way.

Once police found him at 4am walking on the still-busy A1.

Another time he went missing for 24 hours. A mountain rescue team, police helicopters and diving squads were deployed. After a cold night passed, we expected the worst.

He was found asleep on a bench in a nearby garden. In many ways it was a relief when his mobility deteriorated and he was moved to the private nursing home where he now lives.

I know I am not alone in having a loved one depleted by a pitiless disease, but I hope my father's case may serve as a warning to others who face the same dilemma as my brother and I when asked if we wanted to extend Dad's life.

At first, the PEG tube did what everyone hoped – Dad regained weight and a little strength.

But as the months went by, his disease cruelly cantered on.

Last December, he was hit by a series of awful infections. One morning his home called to say he had pulled his PEG out; Ben and I read that as a manifestation of his frustration – especially as the PSP association told me many sufferers do the same. They are, literally, sick of living. Dad just wanted to die.

But he was hauled in and out of hospital; his PEG replaced and his empty life again prolonged. When, last Boxing Day, I visited him, he had such a raking cough I thought he would choke to death.

Ben and I decided enough was enough. It was time to remove the PEG and let him go peacefully.

So, one Friday in January, Ben sat in a meeting at Dad's home with the home's deputy manager, Dad's GP and the community matron and told everyone our wishes. Dad's GP agreed. She said the PEG was keeping him alive unnecessarily.

That weekend passed in a daze. I sat with Mum, contemplating a world without Dad. I knew we had made the right decision – but still I found myself mourning.

On Monday I spoke to his GP, who assured me she would ensure he was comfortable. He was already on morphine and his dose would be upped so he would be peaceful as he slipped into unconsciousness.

Then came the volte-face. Another meeting was called, which I attended. The manageress, absent last time, was present. It seems she, the community matron and the care staff had convinced his GP to change her mind.

Dad's life, it seemed, was now worth preserving. His PEG, I was told, would not be removed because Dad had quality of life and a reason to keep on living.

The truth is, I believe his carers and his GP were acting not out of mercy or compassion but from fear. They are terrified they will face prosecution if they remove the PEG prolonging Dad's life.

His doctor told me it would be morally wrong – and illegal – to take it out. His carers said that because Dad is no longer able to communicate his wishes clearly, it could be construed as assisting his death if it were removed.

Without the support of Dad's GP, Ben and I are powerless to do the right thing by our father.

Dad, by now almost in a permanent vegetative state, is kept alive by a feeding tube. The anger and impotent frustration I feel would make him really sad (if he knew). And what of his carers' claim that Dad has a quality of life worth preserving?

Every time family – or his friends – has visited him over the past eight months, Dad seems to be asleep. His eyes are shut. Sometimes he has weakly squeezed my hand or raised his thumb at half-mast in response to a question.

The only evidence he is alive comes with the hideous coughing fits that threaten to choke him. Yet his carers have told us they have seen him smile, wave even.

As he doesn't do any of this for us, we were sceptical. For years Dad has worn the 'expressionless mask' common in PSP sufferers.

Disturbed and upset, I told the home I found the claims hard to believe. So they offered to video these moments for me.

Four months on, I have yet to see any footage. However, I must say that he is tended with love and kindness at his care home; we have no complaints on that score.

Now, at least once a month, I make the 350-mile round trip from my home in London to Dad's bedside. I am sad my two-and-a-half-year-old son Burt will never know the fun-loving, sporty man his grandad once was.

And when I think of the many indignities Dad's illness has inflicted on him, I hope – really hope – he will not wait long for death.

Today, he will be sitting in his bed or chair, oblivious to this article, the weather or date.

His weight and body mass index are near perfect thanks to the carefully prescribed formula pumped into his stomach.

To what end? The PEG has worked so effectively it has become Dad's life-support machine.

But the quality of life it is supporting has diminished so much that, surely, it is now time to take it out and let nature take its course.'

I still find this sad to read and often reflect on the alternative life Cilla could have lived had we not found this heart wrenching article.

At last, peace finally came to Colin following his long and protracted battle with PSP. Colin eventually passed on the 9th of January 2016, twenty-four days after Cilla and after enduring an overly extended stay in a body no longer recognised by him or his family.

RIP Colin... You gave more than you could possibly imagine.

The published story by Niki was not only extremely brave on her part, but fortuitous to Cilla, since it epitomised a problem we were about to face. Indeed, for us, the timing could not have been any better, and without knowledge of this article, having a PEG (Percutaneous Endoscopic Gastrostomy) surgically fitted was a strong consideration.

Once I had read Colin's story out to Cilla, she remained silent, and about an hour later asked me to read it out again. It was now, after the second reading, that Cilla decided that Colin's fate was not for her. Immediately she made plans for me to add such provisions into her living will. She wanted me to stipulate her wishes in almost every known document we had to hand that would ultimately prevent her from any further suffering. Her doctor was notified, and these details were finally added to her annual review after a consultation with Cilla. This decision was also independently verified by Dr Jenks from the Countess Mountbatten Hospice.

Cilla and I wish to take this opportunity in thanking Niki, her family and *Daily Mail OnLine* for publishing such a life-changing story.

Now, think very carefully about what has been written so far because it is your decision, along with your loved ones, that is more important here than anything else. Neither I, nor Cilla, would want you to decide your own fate based purely on one article, but I will say this loud and clear: *it made a tremendous difference to Cilla!*

With this newfound information to hand, and Cilla's decision made, we were able to concentrate on other things. Although, in my mind, the benefits made from this decision, would come later.

Dark Days Ahead

In November 2015, I became increasingly concerned about Cilla's breathing as it was sometimes laboured and extremely noisy. One warmish evening as I sat in one of Cilla's favourite spots in the garden and located just outside her window – which was always open during the night at her request – I could clearly hear her spasmodic breathing pattern and, what appeared to be, her groaning lightly on the outward breath. In association with this disturbing occurrence, her breathing appeared to be forced and somewhat unnaturally staggered with long silences in between.

I am aware of sleep apnoea due to the fact that my brother Peter has the condition, and this, in my humble opinion, resembled the symptoms. I listened carefully over a period of time, and even recorded it so it could be played back should it be required. My suspicions were immediately reported to the doctors, and I requested assistance in this matter with, perhaps, the possibility of dealing with the condition.

As a result, Cilla received an appointment in the post to attend an NIV clinic at the Southampton General Hospital. (NIV stands for non-invasive ventilation, which assists and researches mechanical means of supported breathing.)

The appointment date was set for Wednesday, the 25th of November at 1:30 pm.

During the visit, Cilla had blood drawn from the inner part of her wrist for analysis. The blood drawn from here gives an accurate level of oxygen in the blood supply based on the condition of the red blood cells. From this, the doctors are able to establish whether there is an issue or not. In Cilla's case, her oxygen levels were good, but the most telling detail came about when I played back the sound recording I had taken earlier. It appeared my theory was correct, and it also transpired that Cilla had, for some time, been physically using her muscles to breathe in a different way than normal. This meant that her diaphragm was not functioning automatically and her body and external intercostal muscles had adapted to her new way of breathing.

Despite this revelation, it was thought that any medical intervention would not improve the quality of her life, so no further action was taken. This did not appear to concern Cilla and she almost seemed pleased by this.

Ten Days

E very carer knew the rules about coughs and colds, which I insisted was a priority element in trust between us all. Any sign of a cough, cold or sniffle then they were, in effect, placed on quarantine leave.

During the afternoon of the **6**th ***of December 2015***, Georgie was showing signs of a developing cold, so I told her to take the week off to recover; there was no way I could expose Cilla to the slightest possibility of any sort of infection, especially respiratory.

The following day, the **7**th, was an important day for Cilla, and one she had been looking forward to for some time. It was the PSP's annual Christmas lunch held in Emsworth, some twenty-one miles away, and was an event Cilla wanted to attend. As per usual, I got Cilla up and gave her her breakfast, but due to circumstances beyond her control, Hannah was unable to make the morning's shower and hair wash. So Cilla and I muddled through, knowing an enjoyable day out, as tiring as it would be for Cilla, was planned for the benefit of her, her friends and fellow sufferers.

The event was organised by Louisa Roberts-West and was always well attended. It gives the carers and sufferers alike an opportunity to meet up and enjoy the splendours of a wonderful Christmas lunch. The Brookfield Hotel & Hermitage Restaurant is ideally suited to people with multiple disabilities, since they have worked hard to make sure accessibility to all parts of the hotel is paramount. Here, nothing was too much trouble, and Cilla found the trip easy since it involved mostly two and three-lane carriageways, which helped our speeds.

Incidentally, Louisa sadly lost her mother Elizabeth to PSP, who coincidentally was the same age as Cilla when she passed. As a result of Louisa's loss, the PSP Association gained a wonderful organiser of events and monthly meetings in Wherwell Village Hall in Andover, Hampshire. These regular monthly meetings were invaluable to Cilla and was the first place she actually met other PSP sufferers. I hold these meetings in such high regard that I continue going to this day.

Anyhow, the day went well – although Cilla did not eat as much as she would have done normally. Even so, I felt sure she'd enjoyed the day and was pleased to see her friends.

At home, Cilla went straight to bed, and I left her there for an extra half hour before getting her up for tea; it was apparent that she was tired, and actually asked to be settled down at 21:10 that night.

The following day, the 8*th*, we settled into our normal routine, although she was, as to be expected, slightly sluggish after her day out. On rising for breakfast, she asked me to assist her into the toilet, which was not that unusual. Lunch was as per expectation, and during the evening, she listened to her favourite soaps before settling at 22:00.

Once more, although tired, the 9*th* came and went without problem – although her needing the toilet was slightly later than the previous day, and recorded at 13:05. At her request, that evening I settled her down ten minutes ahead of her usual schedule... again, not overly odd.

However, after a reasonably good day, and on the night of the *10th of December 2015*, I had cause to be concerned about Cilla's health. Nothing specific, but there seemed to be something wrong, and even though she did not complain or ask for assistance, I suspected a problem.

Due to these trepidations, at 22:19 I dialled 111 and spoke to an operator who considered everything I was explaining. As usual, I had first to explain PSP and the prognosis before stressing several other points. This is because the statutory and pre theoretical questions are somewhat redundant when addressing PSP. You see, if they do not at first understand PSP, then I am afraid, there is every chance of complications.

Eventually, it was mutually agreed that an ambulance crew would be dispatched due to my concerns. Despite my anxieties, the call was not classed as an emergency and the ambulance eventually arrived at 23:20. On arrival, three technicians came in and pondered their options.

As per usual, a full explanation of PSP was needed to bring them up to date, and during their visit, two of them read and studied Cilla's blog; in fact, I actually printed out a copy for them to take.

Cilla was extremely relaxed about all the fuss going on around her, and flashed me the odd '*I am bored, I want to go to sleep*' looks.

Upon examination, there was a limited amount of what they term 'crackling' coming from the lower part of her lungs, her left in particular. As a result, they decided to call for a doctor rather than transport her to the hospital. Meanwhile, they administered 5mg of Salbutamol via a nebuliser and monitored her breathing and pulse. They eventually left just after midnight, safe in the knowledge that a doctor would be calling within a four-hour window.

At 02:35, the doctor arrived and examined Cilla thoroughly. Much to her relief, following the examination, Cilla was allowed to settle down. The doctor confirmed the 'crackling' the ambulance crew had detected and opted to prescribe antibiotics. I was given twenty-one Co-Amoxiclav 500/125mg tabs to administer three times a day.

Meanwhile, Cilla had had enough and had gone to sleep, so I thought that our 09:00 schedule would be the best time to administer the first course.

Since the *11th* and *12th* passed without too much of a problem, I will now jump in time to Sunday the *13th*.

Halfway through lunch, I noticed how slowly Cilla was reacting to eating and asked her if she was Okay. She shrugged and gave me the thumbs-up sign, before refusing to finish the last half of her meal. I then asked if she wanted her pudding, which consisted of a small pot of yoghurt, and today was her favourite: strawberry. Once again, I received the thumbs-up and started to prepare it for her. Halfway through her yoghurt, I asked her if she needed the doctor, and she frowned and gave me a resounding palm out flat of the hand for NO! I accepted and respected her response, but started to become concerned once more about nothing in particular, much like the night of the 10th.

There was something nagging me about her behaviour so I said: *'I'm sorry darling, but I have to be the adult here and I'm going to call for a doctor.'*

There were no objections, but a tiny huff from her as a sign of resignation due to my insistence.

At 14:03, and on the spur of the moment coupled with the previous experience still fresh in my mind, I changed my option by dialling 999 to request an ambulance.

Whilst we were waiting, I wheeled Cilla into the front room and we sat face to face. I apologised to her and explained why I had called an ambulance, even though I was uncertain of my reasons. We held hands and 'talked' for the short duration it took the ambulance to arrive.

The two-man crew listened to me as I explained both Cilla's illness, and what I thought was her problem; but to be fair that was little to nothing.

After an examination, they both agreed that Cilla should be taken to the hospital for observations. I gently assisted Cilla onto the wheeled stretcher whilst having a cheeky little huggle.

For some unknown reason, the ambulance crew had continued their discussions about Cilla's health beyond leaving the house, and they made several radio calls and telephone calls before beginning transportation.

Up and until then, everything seemed quite casual, so what happened next surprised me beyond belief.

I strapped myself into the little companion seat opposite Cilla as they attached an oxygen mask to her. We were now considered an emergency case, and with blues and twos going, it only took about eight minutes for us to reach the Southampton General hospital. During this time I subtly reassured her about what was going on... she remained calm throughout. From the ambulance, we were taken to a room marked Respiratory Unit, where there was a team awaiting her arrival.

If Cilla was worried about the situation, then she was not showing it; alternatively, I was beside myself not knowing what they obviously did.

The team carried out a set of procedures, which included an NIV check before placing an IV into the back of her right hand. During this time, I just stood back and took in every detail I could. The only time I was asked to leave was when a portable X-ray machine was brought to her bedside. On return to the room I craftily looked at the screen, which clearly showed a chest X-ray and immediately became concerned. Unless I was reading it wrong, I could see that both lungs were completely black. I told myself that this could not be the case, and perhaps I had misread it due to the angle of the screen and glare of the overhead lights.

Cilla smiled my way as I came back into the room, and I held her free left hand to show that she was not alone. Throughout, she never complained, and occasionally signed answers to a short question or two.

By now I had contacted my son Adrian, who lives in Tadley, near Reading. His arrival was a relief to me, but how Cilla actually felt from within was beyond me because she remained so calm.

Included in the team performing the essential checks and tests were two young physios from the respiratory unit. Here, they assisted Cilla with removing a build-up of secretions by pummelling various parts of her chest and back, whilst supporting her with a pillow or two. In between each bout, they would use a suctioning machine to remove any excess mucus that was within reach of the suction tube without venturing too far into the throat. Cilla complied with every instruction and acknowledged with positivity, but I got the feeling she was tiring fast.

It was not long before Cilla was allocated a bed in the Acute Medical Unit, section pink, bed 9. It was my understanding that she would spend the night there, and would be assessed overnight as to whether she could come home the following day or not.

I told Cilla I would let her rest and would come back first thing in the morning. Adrian drove me home that night and I eventually prepared a bag of essentials for the following day – just in case.

Monday the *14ᵗʰ*... I arrived at the Acute Medical Unit, only to find that Cilla had been transferred to Ward D5.

It did not take me long to find her, as I could she her shock of blonde hair through an open door in a private side room as soon as I walked onto the ward. Cilla looked tired but was in good spirits, as usual, and as soon as I was close enough, we both reached out and she squeezed my hand firmly.

However, I was later informed that she had not had a particularly good night, mainly due to necessary physio to remove a build-up of fluids on her chest.

Throughout the day, she had a few visitors and, by now, I all but ignored the usual visiting hours and made myself as inconspicuous as I could. We conversed in our usual manner, and once again, Cilla had nothing to complain about or anything negative to say.

Luckily for me, my niece Muna worked at the hospital and was only too aware of what was happening, and what we were going through, since her boss was, coincidentally, Cilla's doctor. The close connectivity to what was going on intuitively helped me understand what lay ahead, although in truth my mind would not connect for at least another twelve hours or so. Of course, Muna could not, and would not, tell me anything in confidence so, at the time, I was just grateful at seeing a friendly face.

At regular intervals, I turned Cilla's pillows due to the amount of sweat she was producing. It was while I was doing this that I remembered Cilla once telling me: **'Horses sweat, men perspire and ladies glow.'**

I smiled at this sudden thought.

Using a baby wipe, I stroked her face and brow as often as I could, and could sense the relief in her face as I did this, so I continued throughout.

We had regular huggles, and it was here that we tacitly reassured each other without a single thought of anything else that was going on in the real world; in truth, the real world was here in the room.

Once more, I headed home that evening, but with a plan in mind to have Cilla transferred home at the earliest opportunity.

Tuesday the *15th* arrived, and my mission was to get to the hospital as soon as I could... but I was certainly not prepared for the information I eventually received on my arrival. The first thing I wanted to do was to poke my head around the door to say hello to Cilla, but was stopped before I could... Dr Emily Heiden had just left Cilla's room following, I guessed, an examination.

My heart sank and I feared the worst since I could read faces... and there were a lot of faces around me showing signs of anguish. I was soon invited by Dr Heiden to follow her, as she had something to talk to me about. Initially, and most frustratingly, all the private rooms were occupied, and my fears were increasing with every step that took me further away from Cilla's room. Eventually, a room was found in an adjacent ward, where I was invited in and offered a seat.

Slowly I sat, with tears already welling up in my eyes, and mindfully pre-empted what I was about to be told.

Dr Heiden could not have been nicer, but nobody could have prepared me for what was to come, as I was told that Cilla had had another bad night. She said that during a particularly tense session of physio she had asked them to stop and to leave her alone.

Apparently, the physios were as close to being as invasive as they could without over-stepping the mark.

This revelation convinced me that Cilla had had enough, since she would normally do anything to help, not herself, but those about her. For her to say, '**Stop!**', must have meant that she knew exactly where she was in the grand scheme of things.

Now came the news I had always been dreading: It had been decided that since Cilla had a DNACPR (do not attempt cardio pulmonary resuscitation) in place, and due to her current refusal of treatment, they were going to take her off her antibiotics.

It was quite clear to me what this meant, so I asked the most obvious question: *'How long?'*

Being so close to Christmas, I was not sure if the answer would make a difference or not, but I swallowed hard and awaited the answer: *'Worst case scenario, two days. At best, two weeks...'*

For the first time since Cilla was diagnosed with PSP and labelled terminal, it all of a sudden felt far too real for me to take in. But then what did I actually expect? Why now was I feeling so vulnerable to the most obvious conclusion the disease had to offer?

Before she left the room, Dr Heiden lifted all restrictions and visitation rights for me, and anybody else who wanted to come and see her. It was this that made me realise exactly how real the situation was, and I felt cold, numb and... selfishly... alone.

Eventually, I was left alone to gather my thoughts, and as unrealistic as it seems, I still hung onto the hope that this was not actually happening. My mind flitted around from one thought to another... some realistic, others not so.

Finally, I pulled myself together and went back to the ward, took a deep breath, and entered her room to resume where we left off the day before. Cilla was brighter than I had hoped, and I soon told her that I had arranged for an array of visitors to come and see her. I could tell by the look on her face that she understood and, once more, she hid her true feelings to prevent me from the pain of what we both already knew and expected.

Unfortunately, up and until now, I'd had great difficulty in reaching Joe, who had recently moved from St Ives in Cornwall to Poole in Dorset. Finally, following message after message left on his answer phone, he contacted me; but due to distance and a lack of transport, Joe was unable to immediately make the journey.

By 10:00 that morning, some of Cilla's visitors had already arrived and it was most telling who had arrived first: Georgie, who had previously been ill with a cold, showed she could not wait to see Cilla, and she was accompanied by another two of Cilla's former carers: Naomi Gibbs and Hannah Ramsey. Soon after, my son Adrian and Hannah Foster arrived – which under normal circumstances was a recipe for fun. Somehow, between them all, they did not disappoint, as Cilla found the strength to laugh at all the stories being relayed. This physically cheered her no end, since now the 'gang' of girls were reliving stories much to the mirth and merriment of them all. Cilla too joined in the best she could, and although she was wearing an oxygen mask she could be heard laughing.

While this was going on, I observed one notable thing: Cilla was virtually unable to raise her hands to acknowledge any questions put her way.

Almost lazily, she would answer by briefly turning her hand and raising it no more than an inch or so off the bed.

As hoped, chaotic scenes soon reigned within the room, and banter prevailed, but unfortunately, like most things, it rapidly came to an end as the girls said their goodbyes and left, leaving just Adrian and me.

Soon afterwards Dr Jenks appeared, and we immediately discussed the possibility of getting Cilla home, where I knew she wanted to be in her final moments. Within an hour, I received a telephone call from a company asking if somebody would be at home the following morning to receive a supply of oxygen. Without question, if this meant Cilla would be able to have her final moments at home, then so be it. Of course, I was warned that the journey home would be the most dangerous time for her, but under the circumstances, I knew she would have wanted nothing more than a fighting chance. Dr Jenks and the other doctors and senior nursing staff were all doing as much as they could to make sure this happened, so I told Cilla; she looked at me and smiled before squeezing my hand firmly.

Later in the early part of the afternoon, Cilla had two other visitors: her brother Paul and a former carer, Rose Jones. As Rose and Adrian chatted to Cilla, I discretely asked Paul to step outside for a talk – although I knew Cilla understood what was going on around her. Paul looked at me knowingly, and gave me more comfort than I could return as my resolve was now breaking down minute by minute.

Paul eventually left, in full knowledge that this might possibly be the last time he would see his little sister; it was now that I recalled the story they had both so enjoyed relaying about his return to Fair Oak all those years ago... sixty-two to be precise.

Soon after this, I took an hour out and left the building before returning just after Rose had left, leaving just Adrian with his '*mum*'. Being mid-December meant early darkness, and I felt the gloom drawing in closer by the second.

By 21:20 that evening, Adrian had left and I dragged a large wing-backed chair as close as I could to Cilla's bed. By placing the bed's folding supports in the down position, I was able to rest my arm on the bed and hold Cilla's left hand. Due to Cilla's perfect nails, it was impossible for a monitoring system to be placed anywhere but on her large right toe, and from where I sat, I watched the electronic SATS (oxygen saturation) readout flash from one end of the spectrum to the other. Her heart rate was fluctuating from as low as forty-five to as high as ninety: even though she was on a direct oxygen feed, her SATS were all over the place.

At 22:00, I turned her pillow and, once more, smoothed her brow with a baby wipe.

By now, the only way we could communicate was through the power of Cilla's hand squeezing mine. In the best way we could, and under the circumstances, we had a huggle... and I told her I loved her before asking if she loved me. She briefly smiled as I received a resoundingly hard squeeze in response. I sat once more, and got up again an hour later to repeat the process. This time, Cilla's eyes were half-open and her breathing was more laboured, despite the hospital's direct oxygen feed. Again I asked her if she loved me as I did her. She had heard me, but only had enough strength to give me the faintest of squeezes, and although faint, it was a recognised response to the question I had just posed.

I continued mopping her brow, although from then on I noticed a clamminess about her and a lack of awareness... I am now convinced that she had slipped into a coma.

As I sat watching the mesmerizing movements of the digital readout, and whilst still holding her hand, I drifted back and forth into sleep. Suddenly, something made me become more alert... I looked at the monitor seconds before it flat-lined and shrieked out a single note... I leapt up and screamed out her name as I looked at her peaceful face, eyes still half-open.

I touched her forehead, as if I was trying to prove that the machine was lying. I also felt for a pulse... *there was none!* It was exactly **01:10** on the morning of **Wednesday the 16th of December 2015.**

She had gone... !

It did not take me long to get two of the night nurses into the room who, in turn, looked at me, then the machine, before repeating the process. Finally, one of them disconnected the monitor as the other removed the oxygen mask, which I had deliberately left on. Cilla took two more of the shallowest breaths I had ever seen taken; although this could have been an automatic and involuntary reaction to the removal of the oxygen mask.

I stayed with her for an hour more, before the on-call doctor arrived to confirm her death.

At about 02:30, and following several telephone calls, I left and slowly made my way back to my car.

My Cilla was gone, but everything about me was still going on: laughter in the background; the sound of people talking in the distance; and the vague hum of traffic hung in the air.

Everything from here on was surreal.

Still Giving

D o you recall me mentioning two very important points earlier when I revealed the details about the living will? Well, this is the second of those points:

In essence, and beyond death, Cilla took one more chance of sticking her middle finger up at PSP, and she took it with both hands held high.

On the 27th of April 2013, Cilla signed a document that was as courageous as it was prophetic: Cilla decided to donate her brain, spinal cord and dura – dura mater or dura is the thick membrane that is the outermost of the three layers of the meninges that surround the brain and spinal cord. Basically, the primary function of the meninges is to protect the central nervous system – to the academically distinguished, Queen Square

Brain Bank for Neurological Disorders at the UCL (University College of London).

https://www.ucl.ac.uk/ion/departments/molecular/ themes/neurodegeneration/brainbank

By due process, documents were signed – and I believe this was the last document physically signed by Cilla – and posted, before being officially acknowledged by the aforementioned department within UCL.

In effect, Cilla had said in advance: *Here is my brain. Do something positive with it towards the cure of PSP.*

Now, thinking back on previous events in her life, I feel there was a semblance of order in Cilla's death, and fate also played its part in the outcome. In essence, Cilla played out her final moments in true style... event by event, and sequence by sequence.

Now, consider this. Had Cilla been at home at the time of her death, then would her final wishes have been realised? Is it possible that there could have been complications and unnecessary delays had she been at home in her final hour? You see, for a brain to be of any worth to the project, then it needs to be removed and preserved within forty-eight hours after death – although this may vary country to country. In this instance, and by 11:30 on Thursday the 17th of December 2015, Cilla's wishes were realised...

I cannot express to you the true worth of somebody like Cilla, who was prepared to give so generously right to the very end. Not only did she forward-plan, she made sure that the plan would work beyond her life. In life, she gave existence, humour, purpose and energy; in death, she left a legacy well beyond human expectation and memories to treasure forever.

Before I move on, I want to remind you of two things: firstly, that I urged you to make a will, and secondly, that Cilla was a great diarist.

By taking the first point now, the second will automatically make sense and which you can adopt.

In making a will, we do not bring forth our end, or accelerate the process. No, what we actually do is give peace of mind to those we leave behind.

Personally, I still find it amazing that people do not take time to complete this simple process that can make such a difference later.

Now for the reason I wanted to raise this point.

As I have told you, Cilla did as much as she could to help in the process of developing this book due to her fantastic foresight. So it should not have come as a complete surprise to me when I found one particular entry in her 1994 diary. Exactly mid-way through the diary was a notes page, which reflected the year so far. Accordingly, I have selected this passage from it:

'My Tao cat is no more, I still hear him in my mind and can feel his warm furry body. He was my last link with Dad and <u>no one</u> knows how much I miss him. I don't talk about it. But I dream of him and wish so much he was still here. Thank God for my wonderful Annie & Emma. I love them far too much. If anything happens to them... well... Oh! no – please not.

I wonder if someone will read this one day, when I'm gone. Is it you Steve? How I loved you my darling. Miss me – don't you? Silly old sod!! Remember how I used to make you laugh. Only remember the happy times, cos they were 99.9% of the time – Honest!!'

There are no words to describe how I felt when I eventually found this entry some twenty-two years' later... and yes, it did catch me by surprise!

Okay, I realise that she was not aware of her impending illness at the time, *BUT*, it does highlight her forward thinking and exceptional perception.

I think if you link the two segments together, you will finally get an understanding of what I am trying to say here. If you have not got the link, then I shall make this point clear one more time: Help your loved ones by helping them understand your future needs, and if you can, write down how you feel now and again. It can... no, strike that... it *will* make a difference!

On a separate note, and as amazing as this sounds, I have two reasons for feeling grateful that Georgie suffered a cold and was given time off.

Firstly, I spent more time with Cilla during that week than any recent other, and secondly, circumstances played into our hands that would have otherwise slipped us by. By spending the extra time with Cilla, I can now look back without regret and in the full knowledge that between Cilla and I, we saw the illness through to the very end... side by side and together!

There is also the strange empathetic feeling I had on Sunday the 13th when I sensed that something was wrong. It is also possible that this connection might not have been made if Georgie had not gone off sick.

Reflections

Cilla's funeral was not, to say the least, traditional at all.

Planned to a 't' she left me very little to do but follow the plan. All I had to do was decide when, where and by whom. Christmas was upon us and within a week thereafter, a New Year loomed without much expectation on my part.

At times like these, we all need support, and that I needed in bucket loads. Fortunately, once again Cilla prevailed and supplied me with an extraordinary amount of support in the form of everybody she had ever touched with her charm. Offers of help and assistance came in all forms... For example, the 'girls' organised the flowers – My sister Joan arranged the food and refreshments –

and Joe provided the memories... many happy memories.

Support also came in the most unusual quarter and one that I was not quite expecting. Through personal recommendation, I chose a local independent funeral director to oversee all aspects of Cilla's final care. Jonathan Terry made the transition so easy that I actually put my grief to one side for a while due to his extraordinary understanding. Furthermore, once it was realised that Cilla had a connection to both Beaulieu and old cars, it was suggested that their immaculately kept 1958 maroon and black Rolls Royce Silver Cloud hearse be used for the occasion.

The date was set for Wednesday the 6th of January and well after the holiday period was over. Cilla would definitely have approved of all of these arrangements because she would not have wanted to mar others festivities... these considerations, I know, would very much be in keeping with her own thoughts.

Between the 16th of December and the 6th of January, everything seemed a blur. The day itself, however, is as crystal clear to me now as it was then. You see, I chose to conduct the service myself, and with the help of Jonathan Terry, my brother Peter and my son Adrian, I was able to concentrate on just that.

The crematorium was packed and people had to find standing room at both the back and down the sides. An estimated one hundred and forty people attended from as far back as her youth, to work colleagues, recent carers and, of course, family.

After a shaky start, I got proceedings underway.

There was love, colour, poetry, music, memories, tears and laughter... much laughter. Cilla generated much of this laughter herself by providing the means for me to relate some of her stories. Indeed, she was instrumental in all aspects of this glorious event since she had fore planned the entire schedule... thus, once more, proving her worth.

Although sections of this might sound slightly macabre, they are not meant to be since we were all there to say goodbye to Cilla and for her to have the best send-off we could offer. With Jonathan's help and from the comments I received later, I think we achieved that.

Also, you may well recall my thoughts about the night of April the 15th when I 'liberated' Cilla's ashes in St Ives... I remain firmly convinced that the send-off we gave her in January was eventually rewarded by her actions in April. By that, I mean the breath-taking experience I felt on the night and the subsequent feeling of total exhilaration was brought on by watching her ashes 'dance' before me as she said a fond farewell.

Incidentally, on that day alone, the PSP Association received donations worth well over £200 in Cilla's name. To those who contributed, I wish to personally thank you since I have not had a chance to find out who donated what since some were anonymous. Thank you!

Cherished Moments

A s this heading is 'Cherished Moments', I have to carefully consider which moments are the most cherished. In truth, this is far too difficult for me to underline with any one defining moment, so I have simplified it to just three.

Firstly, Cilla had a passion for animals, and this is apparent in much of what you have already read. In this instance, I recall the first pet we ever had as a couple: Annie, the Schnauzer. Even now, I have to be careful not to select more of the many hundreds of stories that relate to her, so I will leave it as this! Thomas, our friend from Sweden, had, like Cilla and I, travelled extensively throughout the world. So when one day he asked us what Scotland was like, it made us think. The only possible answer we could give was that we did not know because we had not been there! Later that evening we plotted a round Britain trip, starting from the west coast, and from there, wherever the fancy took us as long as we ended up in Scotland. We had no formal plan, and since Annie was going to come with us, we did not even consider accommodation.

A month later, and with two weeks to kill, we set off. From Lands End to John O'Groats via the west coast.

In Cornwall, Annie was made welcome in one of the smaller bed and breakfasts, so that was where we stayed. The next stop was less inviting so with an estate car, sleeping bags, a quilt and courage, we found a quiet spot and settled there for the night.

The pattern had been set, and Britain shrank as we flitted from one place to the next.

Scotland was everything we ever imagined it to be: friendly, beautiful and mystic. We did everything we could in the short time available to us, which included taking the lift to the furthest reaches of Ben Nevis. Realistically, we were ill-equipped for the ascent, since we were wearing casual, flimsy clothing, so our stay above the clouds was both cold and short lived... but memorable. Annie too felt the cold chill and shivered, despite being tucked under my jacket.

At one point, we decided to stay in a lovely lodge hotel located in the small village of Luss on the bonnie banks o' Loch Lomond. For our added interest, the location was also used in the filming of the television series, *Take the High Road*. It was also here that we visited a shop that produced the various tartans and famous bagpipes.

Before we reached this point, we also stayed on the Mull of Kintyre, made famous by Paul McCartney and his band Wings.

There is also another reason for me to remember our visit to Scotland: Cilla insisted she drive while I rested after a long stint behind the wheel. It did not take me long to realise that this was a mistake since Cilla decided to put her foot down! Her usual driving skills were not something I was particularly worried about, but her speeds were far outreaching the legal limits. Due to this, I insisted I took over the driving for safety's sake. When she final agreed, four miles' later I was pulled over by the police for doing three miles an hour above the legal limit of thirty! Cilla thought this was hilarious, especially since she had reached speeds above seventy when she was driving!

I duly had three penalty points and a fine of £40!

In truth, this did not mar the occasion, and I can honestly say I thoroughly enjoyed our time there.

So, one speeding ticket later, we finally followed the east coast down to Yorkshire. Here, Annie would be walked beyond endurance as Cilla devised a plan, which follows as thus: I was to drive exactly one mile away and park, leaving Cilla and Annie behind to walk following the same route I had just taken. To be fair, and due to the landscape, it was possible to see well beyond a mile, so they knew exactly where I was situated. Anyhow, if Cilla passed the car and carried on walking, then I was to repeat the process. In the end, and after several miles, Annie stopped by the car and refused to walk another step. It appeared that Cilla was enjoying herself so much that it was no longer about walking the dog, it was about relishing life outside the norm.

The second cherished moment is slightly out of sequence, and nearer to the end of Cilla's life. As you already know, we married in the month of September – the 16th to be precise. So, when I heard that *Priscilla Queen of the Desert* was going to be playing at the Mayflower Theatre during this time, I knew exactly what to do.

I was about to book the tickets for the 14th when I realised one important thing: due to the age and structure of the listed building, I knew the disabled seating would be too far back and to one side for Cilla to fully appreciate the show, so rather than go through the normal channels, I decided that the direct approach was the best course of action. I phoned the management team, who helpfully arranged for Cilla and I to sit in the front row where they reserved a certain amount of seats for sight-challenged people. Cilla certainly fitted the criteria, so it was agreed that two front row seats would be reserved in her name. On the night, and with the girls on board, they gave Cilla the works: her hair was coloured with two shades of red and plaited, make-up was applied, and brightly coloured clothes put on; she looked *amazing*.

On arrival, the management went one stage further (again, no pun intended, but, I think by now I deserve this one!) and arranged for one of their staff, Kerry Brady, to be available on the night to assist by any means possible. Kerry kindly provided extra padding for Cilla's seat, and took her wheelchair away for safekeeping.

With the music, atmosphere and brightest of hues in full technicolour, the evening was a complete success.

For safety reasons, we remained in the theatre after the rest of the audience had gone while Kerry retrieved Cilla's wheelchair. As I stood there, I looked around and tried to picture all the shows, concerts and events that had taken place over the years; if the walls could speak, I would have gladly sat and listened to every word.

Anyhow, apart from the fun aspect of the show, and the music, if there was any one defining link to this particular evening and her past, then it was the day Cilla's father dragged her onto the same stage to meet Mr Pastry back in the 1960s.

At the end of the show, and since the evening was still relatively young, I decided to take Cilla on a walk down memory lane. We returned to the car and got everything we needed to make sure she remained warm and comfortable, before I pushed her into town. As I walked, I gave her a running commentary of all the changes the city had recently seen. It was now that I realised most of the changes that had occurred over the years she knew little about. Following a few rests, we eventually reached the precinct, before finishing up by the Bargate. Throughout, I talked constantly about shops, bars and restaurants now gone, and where they once stood. I know she was taking everything in during this time, as her mind was still so active, and I am convinced that during the evening she recalled all sorts of happy memories – some going well back and beyond our thirty-seven years together. At this point in writing, I now wonder if at any stage she recalled her experience with the stalker all those years ago. It is possible, because we passed the very point where the incident occurred.

Anyhow, to top things off, a week or so later we received a note from the star of the show, Duncan James, which also included an autograph.

The note simply read: '*Dear Priscilla, sending you lots of love.*'

I know she appreciated this gesture, and if you could have seen the look on her face when I read the note out then you would fully realise how much it truly meant to her!

Finally, and without doubt, you have by now already learnt that Cilla put her all into everything she did; however, her absolute and enduring love was her garden... so this concluding cherished moment reflects that.

To her, the thought of not being able to maintain the garden filled her with dread. Over the years, Cilla knew I was not much of one for gardening, and even if I were, my priorities eventually changed due to her illness.

By this, I mean that I had to put the garden second to her care, no matter what the circumstances were.

At the time, the garden was furthest from my mind and, as a result, it eventually became a wild haven for all sorts of animals and various other creatures. But it would have to wait, since we had much more important things to worry about. Nevertheless, I felt bad seeing her looking out and towards the wilderness, and even with her failing eyesight and mobility, we both knew she was powerless to do anything about it. At the time, I was not sure what I could do to ease her pain because, by now, it was well beyond mere maintenance and my meagre abilities. Then it struck me: why not turn it into a sensory garden, in which Cilla could hear, touch, smell and, given some strong solar-powered lights, even see?

Fortunately, we were more than blessed to have found the services of a knight in shining armour... Enter Dave Landsey! Dave and his friend Andy stripped the garden bare, and removed every trace of what it had become; but not before saving some of Cilla's most prized plants, trees and shrubs.

Despite the state it was in, the stripping of the garden was not as upsetting or as brutal as it sounds!

I bought eight six-by-six replacement fence panels and nine posts, which Dave soon had in situ. Later, a team of friends and neighbours – Abdul El-Kindy, Chantelle Allen, Dan Nash, Peter Hill and Robin Alsford – laid down a layer or two of weed-suppressing fabric, before six tons of medium-sized shingle was placed and evenly spread, covering the whole garden. A new shed, patio and stone edging were then positioned, before the vast amount of pots Cilla had accumulated were arranged in some semblance of order. This was all planned, designed, and actioned within a one-month period. The finishing touch was a two-tiered fountain with underwater lighting, which gave a beautiful reflective shimmer to the newly painted shed walls. Even the three birdbaths that had been neglected for so long were cleaned and revived ready for use.

With wind chimes, running water, evening lights and the scent of flowers and herbs, Cilla had a brand new garden. A slope was even built to make it easier for her to visit the garden more frequently. As you know, some of the carers freely gave up their valuable time to help make this process happen, as Cilla 'watched' its gradual development.

Initially it was difficult to judge exactly what Cilla thought of my efforts, but she fully understood my sentiments. Due to her now apathetic nature, she rarely expressed facial signs of emotion. However, when I had a chance to take her out there for the first time, she was keen for me to wheel her up the path and around the various features. All in all, I know she was quite pleased, if not more so, with the end results and thanked me and all concerned.

Now, as the summer approaches, I can fully envisage sitting outside on the occasional balmy evening in what is now, in effect, a memorial garden, as the garden now represents someone whose life impacted on all of those who met her over the years... but none more so than mine.

There is a poem that Cilla particularly liked. It is hewn in rock and hangs on the wall of the brick shed in the garden, and is well known to many a gardener.

It reads:

> *The kiss of the Sun for pardon*
> *The song of the bird for mirth*
> *One is nearer to God in the garden*
> *Than anywhere else on Earth*

The poem itself represents Cilla's tribute to her father Douglas, and in different guises, has always appeared in our gardens. I am sure it was her way of thanking her father for giving her the generous gift of gardening.

Her gardening gift to me was an olive tree – currently awaiting a re-pot – and is in pride of place just outside the back door where it can be seen daily.

Laughter was another gift, and something that set Cilla apart... and her exploits over the years reflect this. It is easy to see why so many people fell in love with her, and why she kept friendships going over a vast amount of years.

While not a cherished moment as such – certainly not in the sense of the previous three examples – I do have a memory that I cannot shake from my mind or easily forget.

Although remote, I have decided to include this as a special memory, since it epitomises a process we both experienced but from much different perspectives.

Something occurred one morning when I went into Cilla's room to get her ready for breakfast. Unusually she was still sound asleep when I entered, and appeared to be twitching heavily while moving her feet and arms. Under normal circumstances this commonly indicates a dream is in progress. On closer inspection her eyelids mirrored the twitching, much like one would in REM (rapid eye movement) sleep.

Intrigued, I did not rouse her immediately, and instead sat beside her whilst continually observing her movements. Her legs and feet moved in short jerky movements, as did her arms and hands – like someone running. After a few minutes I gently woke her, before getting her into a seated position.

While she was sitting, I asked her if she still dreamt. She gave me the thumbs-up before I asked another question: *'What were you dreaming about just now?'*

She looked at me blankly for a brief second before telling me, in her own way, that if she was, then she did not recall.

Then I asked the most obvious question: *'Do you still dream as you used to?'*

Her eventual answer soon had me in tears, since it was something I had not thought of up and until then. She indicated that she still dreamt, and that in her dreams she could do everything she could no longer do now. She further explained that she could run, jump, skip, talk, ride horses, and even fly!

One word I have not included in the list of things she could do in her dreams was to laugh. Although in a fashion she could still laugh then, I knew what she meant, and it was this, perhaps, that affected me the most as her laughter was as much her persona as anything else I could mention to describe the very essence of being Cilla!

The tears I mentioned came soon after I had handed her over to the carers, and when I was alone. I do not know why I had assumed that the illness would cause her to suddenly stop dreaming. It stands to reason that if your brain is in perfect working order, then why would dream patterns cease or change? I then imagined what it must feel like being in her position and having these dreams. I now ask you to do the same...

- § -

Stop Press!

Whilst editing this book, I thought the story had come to an appropriate conclusion; however, I was wrong. On the morning of the 8th of April 2016, I received a telephone call from the Queen Square Brain Bank for Neurological Disorders at the UCL (University College London), and although welcome, the call was not expected so soon.

It is important to remember that I did agree, in accordance with section eleven of the consent form, to be kept informed about the findings. If you do consider any form of tissue donation, then take this point into account!

In my case, I wanted... actually, I *needed* to know... everything related and relevant to PSP.

Anyhow, the basis of the call was to inform me that a full neuropathological diagnosis had been carried out on Cilla's brain. The findings were clear, and the pathologist irrefutably confirmed that Cilla had indeed developed PSP.

Though personally, in later life, I think the evidence was conclusive enough.

Due to the highly technical diagnosis, I have only included an easy to understand translation, which, within itself is quiet telling and offers sufficient proof that some progress is being made. Furthermore, it is my personal conclusion that without help from people like Cilla, then the crucial work at the Queen Square Brain Bank for Neurological Disorders would be made much more difficult. Remember, their work cannot take these vital steps forward without our help, consequently, I have also decided to donate my brain since 'healthy brains' are also required for comparison.

Nonetheless, since Cilla wanted nothing to be left out, I wish to share the findings from a letter I received on 12th of April.

With their kind permission, I have, therefore, fully 'incorporated' the covering letter, which I have included to dispel any thoughts that the

Queen Square Brain Bank for Neurological Disorders do anything but take full consideration towards you and your loved ones. I find it both comforting, and reassuring that there are those who are working tirelessly 'behind the scenes' towards both a treatment and a cure of PSP.

7 April 2016

Dear Mr Dagnell

The late Mrs Priscilla Jane Dagnell

Professor Janice Holton has now completed the detailed neuropathological examination of your wife's brain, and has confirmed the clinical diagnosis of progressive supranuclear palsy (PSP).

PSP is a brutal and progressive neurodegenerative disorder for which there is no cure at present. I would like to take this opportunity to express our gratitude to you for your wife's generous donation as this will be of enormous help with our on-going research here at the Queen Square Brain Bank and Sara Koe PSP Research Centre, in our quest to find the cause and treatment for this malady.

If you have any questions, which you think we could clarify, please do not hesitate to contact Karen Shaw, our nurse specialist, at the Brain Bank on 020 7837 8370.

Yours sincerely

Tom Warner

Professor of Neurology

-

Conclusion:

This patient had a clinical history of progressive supranuclear palsy. Histological examination confirms this diagnosis with a typical distribution of neuronal and tau pathology consistent with progressive supranuclear palsy. In addition, there is amygdala predominant Lewy pathology.

Diagnosis:

1. *Progressive supranuclear palsy*
2. *Amygdala predominant Lewy pathology*

Date of report: 22 March 2016

Professor Janice Holton
Professor in Neuropathology

Amazingly, what you have just read, is yet another chapter in Cilla's life, not death since she had the foresight in making arrangements to donate such a vitally revealing organ!

As promised, and with the kind assistance of those concerned at the Queen Square Brain Bank for Neurological Disorders at the UCL, to simplify it all I include the following summary:

'Everyone has tau protein in their brain. When it behaves normally tau protein is essential for the healthy functioning of nerve cells. There are different forms of tau in the human brain and by studying tissue from donors who had a diagnosis of progressive supranuclear palsy in life, we have found a change in a specific form of tau, which distorts the fine balance of cell functioning. Observations of the post mortem PSP brain reveal abnormal accumulations of tau, a clumping together into 'tangles' that clog up the nerve cells leading to their malfunction and eventual loss. Subsequently, and sadly, the loss leads to the symptoms of the disease.

Such abnormal clumping of different proteins is now recognised as a primary cause of several neurological disorders, and great emphasis is being placed on possible therapeutic approaches that prevent or clear this clumping.'

As I have said on many occasions, Cilla wanted you to know everything, and I do not think that this could possibly be any more informative than anything you have already read about her life.

I wish to further emphasise my gratitude to all of those concerned at the Queen Square Brain Bank for Neurological Disorders at the UCL. In particular, for their kind responses to my requests for this detailed analysis. In truth, with their dedicated help I have found this aspect of conveying an understandable synopsis much easier.

- § -

Remember the title?

You... By now, as a reader, I fully expect you to completely understand the intellect and person portrayed within the pages of this book. Everything about her has been exposed to scrutiny, and is without regret. It is up to you to decide how you feel about these revelations, and there is no compunction on *our* part to sway how you feel about the subjects and disclosures within – These are yours to decide.

Me... Cilla, was the 'complete package', and there is nothing more I can add to what has already been written, apart from the final thoughts at the end.

& PSP... the illness – its pattern – its relentless conclusion. I hope you now have a better understanding of how it works and how it will affect sufferers.

I deeply respect what you are going through, and hope you forgive some of the brutality within the transcript... However, I make no apologies for the reasons behind them.

- § -

Despite everything that happened to Cilla over the years – especially when she became bedridden – she decided that it would be for the best if her friends remembered her as she was, and not what she had become.

Of course, we all have our own memories of her but I now ask you, please remember Cilla as she asked to be remembered!

Finally, do you remember the question Cilla asked herself only once? Well, I have asked that self-same question on her behalf every day since: *PSP... Why Cilla?*

I think it is fair to say that you have read a whole life's story spanning 66 years from start to finish. In doing so, you have been added to the list of people who now keep Cilla's memory going... Thank you for reading.

RIP Cilla x
23.07.1949 – 16.12.2015

About The Author

*S*teve Dagnell – aka – *Shelby Locke* was born and raised in Southampton, UK where he still lives. Educated in the state school system, he confesses that his schooling was nothing more than ordinary. Although he enjoyed his time there, he declares, *"Going to school was, for me, sometimes problematic. Looking back, I believe that in life, it is what you learn beyond this point that makes a difference. The disparity I am talking about is based on the much quoted school of 'hard knocks', and how to survive them beyond today"*.

Being dyslexic, and hard knocks aplenty, he survived not knowing the alphabet until the age of nineteen! Although he could read and write, once he understood the basics in English he then turned to word puzzles. His first attempt at crosswords helped him understand words and how they fitted into sentences. Somehow, and with the help of his wife Cilla, he expanded his understanding of literature and soon began to experiment with poetry. Poetry was quickly left behind in favour of conventional stories.

In 2010 he turned his sights on Novels. He wrote his first, based on local history, and what turned out to be a well-documented International disaster. The ill-fated liner *Titanic* features strongly in his first novel *'Stepping'*. Using a combination of fact and fiction, he has been able to put together a *'rip roaring story'*, which takes the reader through an *'amazing journey'*. By applying his imagination, he has come up with a *'unique yarn'* combining several time lines.

'Stepping Back', is the final instalment of the set and, although connected, the story takes you on a completely separate path. This path links directly to some of the characters in *'Stepping'*, by showing how things could be different in an alternative everyday life.

'One for Rose Cottage', Rose Cottage and Claire Chambers are inextricably linked! Rose Cottage holds a secret, and Claire Chambers is the only person who can reveal the mystery that surrounds it! She has been chosen to 'open a door', which

some would rather leave closed and are prepared to do almost anything to keep it that way.

Claire now walks a path others have trodden, and have not survived unscathed. The path is littered with broken hearts, dreams and lives... For some, there cannot be peace until the final mystery is solved and Claire must find a way to do this without being drawn into a situation where the path has no way back.

All is not as it seems at Rose Cottage and nor will it be until the bitter and bloody end!

The story, or should I say stories, do not stop there! *Several other books are in the pipeline – Look out for 'Marnie Smith'.*

'You, Me & PSP' has given Steve a chance to keep promises made by him to his beloved wife Cilla.

Finally, there are no words to describe this stage of mourning, since each case is immeasurably different. However, by reading this book, you have taken the first steps in trying to understand the process that eventually leads up to a very personal loss.